PATIENT
TEACHING
IN NURSING
PRACTICE

A Patient and
Family-Centered Approach

PATIENT TEACHING IN NURSING PRACTICE

A Patient and Family-Centered Approach

Barbara W. Narrow, R.N., Ed.D.
Syracuse University School of Nursing

A WILEY MEDICAL PUBLICATION
JOHN WILEY & SONS
New York • **Chichester** • **Brisbane** • **Toronto**

65779

Library of Congress Cataloging in Publication Data:

Narrow, Barbara W
    Patient teaching in nursing practice.

(A Wiley medical publication)
Bibliography: p.
Includes index.
    1. Patient education.   2. Nurses and patient.
I. Title. [DNLM: 1. Nurse-patient relations.
2. Patients—Education—Nursing texts. WY87 N234t]
RT90.N37   610.73   78-10241
ISBN 0-471-04035-5

Printed in the United States of America
10 9 8 7 6 5 4 3 2 1

To Wilbur

Preface

This book will help nurses prepare for patient teaching by giving them a conceptual framework and a practical guide for using it.

Some educators believe a very heavy theoretical base should underlie or accompany early teaching experiences, but I believe these experiences will be more successful and satisfying if the reader is helped with the application of a more modest array of theoretical concepts. If a reader discovers that a basic conceptual framework helps her teach, she will want to learn more about the theoretical bases for teaching and learning. Therefore, in accordance with my own philosophy and style of teaching, I have presented theoretical constructs in such a way that the nurse can understand and apply the essence of the theory to her actual nursing practice. The annotated bibliography will enable the reader to study in greater depth the topics introduced in this book. I expect that while a few readers will pursue these selections concurrently with their nursing programs, many more will do so after graduation, as motivation increases with greater involvement in patient teaching and health education.

I believe that the author of a textbook is first and foremost a teacher whose primary responsibility is to synthesize the essence of ideas and theories into a meaningful whole for the reader. The language of this book is simple and direct, so that the time and energy the reader might expend trying to translate an author's rhetoric into understandable phrases may instead be spent integrating the concepts into her own frame of reference.

The purposes of this book are:

1. to help the reader acquire a conceptual framework for the process of patient teaching;
2. to help the reader view patient teaching as an integral part of nursing practice;
3. to present the content in such a way that the reader will feel curious, challenged, and motivated to test the ideas and concepts;

4. to provide the reader with practical ways to use the educational tenets and concepts presented;
5. to help the reader begin to find such satisfaction in patient teaching that she will become committed to a lifelong pursuit of increased effectiveness in patient teaching.

Although this book was written primarily for undergraduate nursing students, I believe that many staff nurses will find it useful, and that students and staff in other health fields will be able to apply the underlying concepts to their own teaching activities.

Finally, I should like to note that, in an attempt to insure simplicity and clarity, I have consistently referred to the nurse as *she* and the patient as *he* with no intention whatsoever of discriminating in any way against male nurses and female patients.

Barbara Narrow

Acknowledgments

I am deeply indebted to my graduate students, because many of the ideas in this book are the direct outcome of insights gained from their honest inquiries and our mutual exploration of important issues.

I would like to thank Kathleen Fitzgerald, R.N., M.S., whose assistance was invaluable throughout the preparation of the manuscript and who demonstrated her concern for patient teaching by making suggestions that have significantly enhanced numerous portions of the book.

I am especially grateful for the interest and support of Cecilia F. Mulvey, R.N., M.S., whose commitment to systems theory, health, and families was exemplified in her comments and suggestions as she meticulously reviewed the manuscript from her perspective as a community health nurse.

B. N.

Contents

PATIENT
TEACHING
IN NURSING
PRACTICE

A Patient and
Family-Centered Approach

PART I

CONCEPTS BASIC TO TEACHING AND LEARNING

1

Teaching, Learning, and This Book

You have been learning from other people since you were very small, often without being specifically taught. You learned how to cut with scissors, how to please the teacher, how to dress like your peers, and how to get along with an irritable neighbor.

In similar fashion, people learn from you, day in and day out, by watching you and listening to you talk. Although they are learning, you are not necessarily teaching, because much of the time you are not even aware of the process. Although there are many ways to define teaching, for the purposes of this book we will consider teaching to be a deliberate, intentional action that is undertaken to help another person learn to do something he presently cannot do.

The fact that teaching, as we have defined it, is deliberate and intentional does not mean that it must be a lengthy or complex task. It *does* mean that you respond with a conscious action to another person's need to learn. It may be that you are responding to a person's verbal request, a puzzled look, a gesture of defeat, or tears of frustration. Whatever the cue, you recognize it as an indication of a need to learn, and in response, you consciously try to help the person learn whatever he needs to know. Sometimes, it may take only a moment or two, but it is a deliberate action on your part; you are teaching. At other times you may need to prepare for days before you attempt to teach a certain person or group. But whether your teaching is spontaneous or planned well in advance, whether it takes two minutes or an hour, whether you are teaching one person or 75, you are engaged in the deliberate, conscious, intentional process of teaching.

It is reasonable to conclude that teaching is done by a teacher, and throughout this book I will assume that the teacher is a person. An educational film, filmstrip, textbook, or tape represents a deliberate effort to teach, but the learning that follows is the result of intentional actions on the part of a human teacher.

The relationship between teaching and learning has been discussed and debated for many years. The question, "Has the teacher taught if the learner has not learned?" is akin to the question, "If no one was there to hear a tree fall in the forest, was there any sound?" In some academic situations it may be appropriate to state that a person "did a fine job" of teaching a certain class despite the fact that a number of students failed to learn. Within the context of this book, however, I am assuming that you have not taught if the patient has not learned. The success of your teaching is measured, not by how much content you have imparted, but by how much the person has learned.

Based upon the above assumption, this book is designed to help you teach by answering the following questions:

What factors influence a person's readiness to learn?

What can you do to increase the likelihood that your patient or client learns whatever you are trying to teach?

How can you tell when a person has learned something?

TEACHING: WHAT IT IS AND WHAT IT ISN'T

Teaching is the process of facilitating learning. It is an interaction designed to help a person learn to do something he is currently unable to do. The thing to be learned may be called an objective, goal, or purpose, but whatever the term, it indicates the nature and focus of the learning. Occasionally, the objectives are set by either the patient or the nurse; in most instances of effective learning, however, the objectives are developed by patient *and* nurse working together.

Teaching is but one aspect of the teaching-learning process, and it is an artificial separation to speak of either teaching or learning in isolation. Teaching is part of a two-way interaction, and in general a one-way communication is *not* teaching per se but is one of the many activities of teaching. For example, telling is NOT teaching, although it may be an important teaching activity. Giving directions, information, or advice is *not* teaching but is an integral part of teaching. Teaching is a process similar in many respects to nursing process, which will be described in a subsequent chapter.

LEARNING: WHAT IT IS AND WHAT IT ISN'T

Learning means that a person becomes capable of doing something he could not do before. Learning includes a wide range of behaviors, from motor skills to intellectual skills. A person is said to have learned when he can explain, discuss, demonstrate, make, or prepare something by using some set of ideas and/or motor skills.

In some settings a person is said to have learned when he is able to do a specified action; in others he is said to have learned when he actually does what he is capable of doing. A math teacher who has taught a learner to solve algebraic equations may be considered an effective teacher even if the learner never again exhibits any interest in algebra. Within the context of health care, however, teaching effectiveness depends upon whether or not the learner actually uses his newly acquired knowledge or skill. I could not say that a nurse's teaching was effective if a patient who had been instructed before surgery how to cough, turn, and deep breathe did not do so after surgery. We could say that he had been *told, instructed,* and *shown* how to cough, turn, and deep breathe. We could agree that he may have understood the nurse's words and that, when free of pain or discomfort, he may have been able to return the nurse's demonstration. It may even have been noted on the patient's chart that preoperative teaching was "done." But what are we to conclude about the teaching-learning process if the patient develops postoperative respiratory complications because of his failure to cough, turn, and deep breathe after surgery?

Throughout this book I will place heavy emphasis upon the behavior of the patient as an indicator of successful teaching. I realize that some patients seem to be difficult, ornery, and apparently unwilling to learn. Every teacher experiences a few failures, and so will each nurse. Some patients cannot be taught within the very real limits of the nurse's time, energy, and patience. The majority of patients, however, are eager to learn the things that they feel are relevant and useful.

The goal of the nurse is to teach in such a way that the patient actually does those things that will contribute to his well-being, to his physical and mental health. Merely knowing *how* to do something has little effect upon one's health; it is the doing that makes a difference.

THIS BOOK: WHAT IT IS AND WHAT IT ISN'T

This book was written as an introduction to some of the theories related to the processes of teaching and learning. It is intended to help you apply some basic concepts related to theories of Carl Rogers, Abraham Maslow, systems analysis, nursing process, and other theories. This book is not intended to be an in-depth reference source for any of these theories. A few concepts that are basic to the teaching-learning process are explained briefly as background for nurses and students whose preparation to date has not included the theories that are essential to an understanding of the focus of this book. The references for each chapter will enable you to pursue in greater depth the topics presented in that chapter.

This book *will not* give you the content for patient teaching that is specific to a given client's condition or situation. This book *will* help you with the process of teaching, with the approaches and methods that will make your teaching more effective, but your textbooks, professional journals, and other reference materials will continue to provide the content of your teaching.

THE BIBLIOGRAPHY: WHAT IT IS AND WHAT IT ISN'T

Two books for the price of one! That's what you get if you use the bibliography of a book. The references in this book will provide access to a body of knowledge equal to that which could be found in a book of selected readings or an anthology of articles related to patient teaching. The content of these references was not included in the text of this book because I feel that it is a waste of time and energy to write again that which has already been well written and published, as long as it is still readily available to the learner at no expense. I do feel, however, that it is a teacher's task to help the learner select useful references from the mass of material in print, and I feel that a carefully selected and annotated bibliography can do this.

The bibliography in this book is not exhaustive; it is not a complete listing of all available references. It is a highly selective listing of articles that either supplement or complement each chapter. In an effort to make the bibliography as useful to you as possible, only those articles that seemed to be especially informative or illuminating have been included. Any "nice to know, but not necessary" or merely "interesting" articles were omitted.

Suggestions for Using the Bibliography

1. As you read each chapter, note the ideas or questions you would like to pursue or study in greater depth.

2. Read over the bibliographic entries for that chapter, and check any references that interest you.
3. Except in unusual circumstances, don't make a trip to the library for only one or two references. It is likely to be an inefficent use of your time. Wait until you have a number of articles to read.
4. To save time, list the references you want to read on a slip of paper, chronologically by journal, *not* alphabetically by author. For example:

    AJN Dec 75 DeBerry p. 2191
    AJN Jan 76 Friedland p. 59
    AJN May 76 Long p. 765
    Can. Nurse Oct 72 Park p. 38
    Can. Nurse Nov 76 Bolevert p. 26

    I find that I can waste considerable time and energy seesawing from one set of journals to another with an alphabetized list of readings, and that the few minutes spent preparing an efficient list is saved many times over.
5. As you read each article, look for relationships between the contents of the article and the book. Each article was carefully selected to expand, supplement, or illustrate the material in a specific chapter or to present a different point of view on the topic.
6. Many of the articles are applicable to several chapters or topics. Whenever a choice had to be made, I assigned the article to the chapter that seemed most directly related to that reference. If several chapters seemed equally appropriate, I usually assigned the article to the chapter with the least number of readily available references. You may not agree with my placement of reference materials, and for this reason all references are grouped into a single bibliography. With references all in one place, it will be easier for you to skim the list to find those that may be useful to you, especially if you plan to use them in a slightly different context. For example, I have grouped all references in terms of the processes of teaching and learning, but you might want to go through the references to find material related to a specific situation, such as teaching adolescents or persons with cardiac conditions.

My criteria for the bibliography of this book were: a) the articles would be useful and applicable to teaching situations likely to be encountered by a staff nurse in almost any setting, b) the majority of articles would be readily accessible to students and staff nurses, and c) the bibliography would be annotated to help you choose references that are relevant to you, since it is impossible to accurately assess the contents and focus of the article from the title alone.

SUMMARY

This book is designed to help you integrate patient teaching into your nursing practice, to introduce some of the theories that are basic to patient teaching, to help you find practical ways to apply these theories, to encourage you to try and test the ideas and concepts that are presented, and—hopefully—to stimulate a lifelong interest in patient teaching.

2

An Overview of
Patient Teaching
What? Who? Where?
When? Why?

WHAT IS PATIENT TEACHING?

Much confusion and many problems surround the use of the term *patient teaching*. These difficulties hamper our communication within the profession about one of the most critical of all nursing interventions, teaching.

There seem to be at least two facets to the controversy: the identification of the learner and the description of the content. Problems related to the identification of the learner arise because the nurse teaches people other than the patient. She teaches relatives, friends, and neighbors of the patient. She teaches groups of people in the community, and she may participate in teaching the general public via mass media. There seems to be no single word to identify the person being taught that is acceptable to the various groups that advocate the use of either *learner*, *client*, or *patient*. The majority of any all-encompassing terms and phrases sound awkward and cumbersome.

Rather than expend time and energy on semantics, throughout the remainder of this book I will refer to the recipients of the nurse's teaching efforts as patients, with the expectation that you will accept this usage as a form of shorthand, and that you will substitute the word of your choice for the word *patient*. The concepts related to teaching and learning that are presented in this book are applicable to any situation, whether the nurse be teaching an individual, family, or group within the community. Furthermore, the concepts basic to teaching and learning are not affected by the word or label that is used to designate the person being taught.

The use of the term *patient teaching* is also controversial because of the content and purposes of the teaching. Since the word *patient* has traditionally been applied to a sick person, the term patient teaching seems restrictive to some nurses, who feel that it does not include health education. There are certainly identifiable differences in the teaching and learning that occurs at each end of the health-illness continuum, but I would suggest that these differences are very quickly obliterated as the center of the continuum is approached. It seems artificial and unnecessary to fret about the semantic differences in most teaching situations. Carried to an extreme, the differentiation between patient teaching and health education could mean that a nurse might be engaged in both patient teaching and health education within a five-minute interval with the same person if the focus and emphasis of the interaction shifted from a recent or present illness to future health. I acknowledge the significance and implications of these distinctions, and the need for such differentiation in those situations in which it is essential, but within this book the term patient teaching will include the promotion of health as well as the prevention and treatment of illness.

And so, to answer the question, "What is patient teaching?" for the purposes of this book, patient teaching is the process of helping a person to learn those things that will enable him to live a longer and/or fuller life, and helping him learn how to reach his optimal level of physical and mental health.

WHO TEACHES THE PATIENT?

The nurse may be viewed as the primary health teacher, but many people contribute to the process of patient teaching. These contributors include doctors and other members of the health care team, friends, families, former patients, and various agencies.

Within the health care delivery system, the extent and type of teaching done depends upon the role and qualifications of each individual. The teaching of the doctor and nurse differs from that of the aide or volunteer worker, yet each contribution can serve a purpose and meet a need. This is true to the extent that all teaching efforts are planned and coordinated. It is not true when teaching is done by default, when an unprepared person teaches what prepared personnel fail to teach. If the professional staff in a clinic or agency gives the appearance of being busy, rushed, or unconcerned, the patient may resort to seeking information from the maid or a volunteer who seems to have time to talk. The information thus obtained is often helpful, but the circumstances under which it was sought represent a serious indictment of nursing responsibility and accountability.

Neighbors, spouses, parents, and grandparents are effective teachers. In fact, the advice and teaching of a respected lay person may at times be heeded more quickly than the teaching of a professional person, especially if ethnic values, folklore, or tradition are involved. These people are aware of the patient's value system, life style, fears, and aspirations, and their teaching is likely to be direct and relevant. The nurse must expend considerable effort and energy to teach in a manner that is equally relevant and meaningful.

Former patients are able to teach new patients effectively, partly because of their empathy and understanding, and partly because of their enthusiasm and interest in helping another person learn to live with a given condition or disease. Examples of organized teaching by former patients are the Ostomy Clubs and the Reach to Recovery Programs for women who have had a mastectomy.

Some agencies have extensive teaching functions. The American Cancer Society is a notable example with its posters, films, television commercials, printed matter, teaching days, and so on. Other examples include the American Lung Association and the March of Dimes.

All of these individuals and groups have something to contribute to the health and welfare of patients and their families, but the nurse is potentially the most significant teacher because of factors related to knowledge, opportunities for teaching, and the nature of the patient-nurse relationship.

First, the nurse has greater knowledge of matters related to health and illness than the nonprofessional persons who interact with the patient, and therefore she has a greater potential for facilitating significant learning, especially if she uses the concern and interest of friends and family to foster the patient's desire for health.

Second, the nurse often has more opportunities for patient teaching than other professional members of the health care team. She spends more time with the patient and is in a position to note both his need to learn and his readiness to learn. The teaching of the nurse is likely to be more intentional and systematic than that of other individuals. Neighbors, family, and friends, as well as many professional persons, are likely to teach only in response to an obvious or urgent need. The nurse, through the use of nursing process, is able to respond to current teaching needs and at the same time provide anticipatory teaching and guidance.

Third, the nurse is able to individualize her teaching and make it relevant to a given patient in a way that is not feasible for most large resource groups. The American Cancer Society cannot teach an individual in the same way that an interested nurse can. Fortunately, patient teaching is not an either-or situation. Both the nurse and the American Cancer Society have special functions, and hopefully the patient and his family can receive the benefits of both. The patient who is learning to live with cancer and the aftermath of therapy needs the support and services of the Cancer Society, and yet a one-to-one interaction with his nurse is probably his most urgent teaching need.

Finally, nurses teach because teaching has long been accepted as an integral part of nursing practice and is now mandated by law in a number of states. Teaching is not an optional activity; it is an essential nursing intervention. With increasing frequency the nurse, in conjunction with the doctor, will be held accountable for teaching the patient and will be liable for failure to do so.

WHERE ARE PATIENTS TAUGHT?

Patient teaching may take place, literally, anyplace, from an intensive care unit to an auditorium, from a laundromat to the patient's kitchen, from a classroom to a summer camp. Teacher and learner may be physically together or may be linked through the media of newspapers, magazines, television, or telephone. Patients may be taught wherever a person who needs to know something comes in contact with a person who knows.

WHEN DOES PATIENT TEACHING OCCUR?

The activities of teaching may take place at any time, but learning occurs only when the patient is ready to learn. At other times he may politely listen, and may even memorize some factual material, without learning anything that will help him to improve his health or well-being.

For the hospitalized patient, there are at least three times in which there is likely to be a concentrated period of teaching. These are: 1) upon admission, 2) at the onset of tests or therapy (including pre- and postoperative teaching), and 3) upon discharge. These are valid times for concern about the patient's needs, but they are not necessarily the most appropriate times for effective teaching. The patient's stress level may be so high at these times that he may be unable to do more than look attentive and listen politely. You can probably remember an instance when your own doctor explained something to you in full detail, and yet, as you left the office, you realized "I can't remember a thing he said."

In time of great stress, the nurse needs to help the patient meet his most basic needs. He needs to learn those things that will help him cope with his current situation; a time of great stress is not an appropriate time for extensive teaching. When the patient is anxious and tense, the very direct activities of explaining, demonstrating, showing, and informing are useful in helping him become physically and psychologically comfortable with at least minimal control over his own situation. The optimal times for more extensive teaching occur when the patient is as physically comfortable and psychologically relaxed as possible, and when he needs to learn how to do something that seems desirable to him. Many nurses use the phrase, "the teachable moment." Unfortunately, this seems to imply that the occasions for teaching are fleeting and spontaneous. In reality, some opportunities for teaching do arise spontaneously, but many are created by the nurse. The skilled teacher recognizes and uses those occasions when the learner is anxious, eager, or "dying" to learn, but she is thoroughly capable of *creating* a situation in which the patient can and will learn those things that he deems important for his well-being. The nurse's sense of timing is critical. The mother who is fatigued by the care of a colicky infant, a lively toddler, or a sick husband may not seem very teachable to a public health nurse who is determined to teach her about immunizations on a given visit. That same mother may be very eager to learn at another time, when she is not so tired or distracted.

WHY ARE PATIENTS TAUGHT?

Very simply, a patient is taught because he has a need and a right to know those things that are relevant to his condition, disease, or situation. There has been a rapidly escalating concern for patient teaching and health education, especially since the American Hospital Association published the Patient's Bill of Rights in 1972. The Nurse Practice Acts of several states now designate patient teaching as a function of nursing; consequently, it is becoming a legal responsibility as well as a moral and professional one.

The purposes or goals of patient teaching may be divided into three major categories: to promote health, to prevent illness, and to cope with illness. These categories often overlap, and in the literature finer distinctions are made, but for the purposes of this book the three major categories will be used.

Teaching to Promote Health

This category includes all teaching that helps to improve the quality of life, facilitates optimal physical and psychological growth and development, increases self-esteem, and promotes self-actualization. Examples of such teaching would include teaching a young mother about the importance of sensory stimulation for her infant, teaching a family about the relationship between communication patterns within the family and the mental health of each member, and teaching a group of parents about the significance of each stage of growth and development.

Teaching to Prevent Illness

This category of teaching helps to eliminate or reduce preventable illness, discomfort, and misery. Examples of such teaching range from genetic counseling in an effort to prevent inherited disease conditions and traits to helping people reduce stress in order to decrease the possibility of stress-related illnesses such as ulcers and hypertension. Other examples might include efforts to prevent obesity, drug abuse, and adolescent pregnancies in which the risks are high for both mother and baby.

Teaching to Cope with Illness

The patient and his family need to learn how to participate in the prescribed nursing and medical regimens, and how to live with a condition that cannot be cured or relieved. The patient and family may need to learn how to promote satisfying interactions with a dying person, how to live with the residual paralysis of a stroke, how to prevent complications such as infection or contractures, or how to cope with problems such as mental illness, alcoholism, child abuse, or mental retardation.

PREREQUISITES FOR PATIENT TEACHING

Some patient teaching is done by nurses who have had specialized training. The patient who is to have home hemodialysis, for example, needs to be taught by a nurse who is experienced in both using and teaching the complex procedures that are involved. Other teaching can be done by any nurse who is willing to do three things: 1) acquire the essential knowledge, 2) develop skill in teaching, and 3) explore with the patient what the condition or situation means to him and his family. There is no substitute for knowledge, skill, or caring, and effective patient teaching demands all three.

3

Systems Theory and Nursing

The familiar phrase, "No man is an island," written over three hundred years ago by John Donne, is a beautiful and poetic expression of today's systems theory. Although Donne never heard of the theory as such, with its crisp and technical vocabulary, he both felt and understood the essence of the concepts. The following passage, taken from one of his *Devotions*, might be described as a vision of the theory that was to follow three centuries later.

> No man is an island, entire of itself; every man is a piece of the continent, a part of the main; if a clod be washed away by the sea, Europe is the less. . . . Any man's death diminishes me, because I am involved in mankind. And therefore never send to know for whom the bell tolls. It tolls for thee.

Current systems theory, in language that is dull by comparison, states that:

1. A system, whether it be a digestive system, political system, heating system, or family system, is composed of a number of identifiable, interrelated parts called components.
2. Since these parts or components are interrelated, whatever happens to one part affects in turn one or more of the other parts, and also affects the overall functioning of the system.
3. Each system is a component of a larger system, and whatever happens to one system affects one or more of the other component systems, and also affects the overall functioning of the larger system.
4. Since all systems are interrelated, the boundaries between systems are established arbitrarily at any given point in time.
5. The functioning of a system is dependent upon the quantity and quality of its input, output, and feedback.

Systems theory has been widely utilized by disciplines such as engineering for a number of years, and has rather recently begun to be applied to various aspects of nursing practice. Since a theory can be of little practical use until it is made operational, that is, until it can easily be applied to everyday situations, the paragraphs that follow will briefly explain the basic concepts of systems theory within the context of the health care delivery system and then apply them specifically to patient teaching.

1. *A system is composed of a number of identifiable, interrelated parts called components.* Nurses are familiar with the systems of the human body, with the parts of each of these systems, and with the relationships of one part of a system to the others. These parts or components are easily identified and described. For example, the mouth, esophagus, stomach, intestines, and rectum are all parts of the digestive system. In other systems, especially the larger social systems, the components are less obvious. The hospital system, for example, is composed of many departments (components), some of which are almost unknown to the nurse and patient. These components of the hospital system include the following departments: nursing, dietary, laundry, medical, laboratory, maintenance, bookkeeping, legal, public relations , and many others.

2. *Since the parts of a system are interrelated, whatever happens to one part affects one or more of the other parts, and also affects the overall functioning of the system.* If a person has all his teeth extracted in preparation for getting dentures, the process of extraction will temporarily affect all parts of his mouth. The resultant inability to chew will affect all parts of his digestive system as well as the overall functioning of the digestive system.

Just so, whatever happens within the hospital laundry affects other parts of the hospital system. If the supply of hot water should fail, the laundry would be unable to supply fresh linen, nurses and aides would be delayed in meeting patient needs, the housekeeping department would be unable to make up fresh beds for new admissions to the hospital, and so on. As serious as these immediate and obvious effects might be, the overall effect on patient care would be even more serious. Such disruption in routines, procedures, and schedules would most likely result in short tempers, frustration, and irritation among hospital personnel, which in turn could create anxiety, discomfort, and other negative responses within patients, families, and visitors. There is no way in which the effect of inadequate hot water can be confined to the laundry. Even if the hospital were able to secure an adequate supply of linen without delay from a commercial laundry in order to prevent the disruption of patient care, the unplanned expense of doing so would affect the budget, bookkeeping, and auditing departments.

3. *Every system is a component of a larger system, and whatever happens to one system affects one or more of the component systems, and also affects the overall functioning of the larger system.* Every clinic, nursing home, doctor's office, and hospital is a system that is a component of the local health care delivery system. This larger system is a component of a regional system, which in turn is part of the state health care delivery system, and some portions of the state system are parts of the federal Medicare system and/or the Department of Health, Education, and Welfare. These interrelationships are complicated and tend to become less obvious as the systems become larger. The individual patient and nurse may be unaware of the relationships, but both are vitally affected by them. For example, any new state regulation relating to standards of care for premature infants will affect the size and type of newborn care facilities in local hospitals, which will affect the number and qualifications of nurses employed, which will in turn affect the rates paid by private citizens, welfare departments, and insurance companies.

4. *Since all systems are interrelated, the boundaries between systems are established arbitrarily at any given point in time.* The setting of boundaries makes it possible for a person or group of persons to work with a single system—to develop it, study it, evaluate it, treat it, or change it. The internist knows that the stomach is a component or subsystem of the digestive system, but he may choose to arbitrarily set boundaries that enable him to focus on the stomach as a system. In another patient, boundaries may be set that enable him to study the interaction of enzymes within the digestive system.

Boundaries are set in accordance with the purposes of the persons working with a system. For example, in order to study the nursing care of surgical patients in hospital X, an initial boundary would be set to include surgical patients and to exclude all other patients at hospital X. The boundaries can then be readjusted to either include or exclude orthopedic surgery, pediatric surgery, neurosurgery, and other specialties. The boundaries might be set to include only adult patients with abdominal, cardiac, or chest surgery. The essential components of the system for delivering nursing care to these patients are the surgical patients themselves and the nurses. If the nurses feel that their nursing care is adversely affected by inadequate staffing, the boundaries must be extended to include those persons in nursing administration who are reponsible for staffing the surgical units. If it seems that the quality of care is related to problems of chemotherapy, the boundaries of the system must be reset to include representatives of the pharmacy department and also the physicians who are writing the orders for the drugs in question.

Another study might be undertaken to examine the care of all surgical patients of all ages and all types of surgery in all hospitals in the county in order to find ways to reduce the incidence of postoperative infections. The boundaries of this large system would include the patients, nurses, infection control consultants, and possibly a statistician. These boundaries are, of course, intangible. They are probably unknown to anyone except those persons who are working with the system, and these arbitrary boundaries do not usually affect the workings of the system in any noticeable way.

5. *The functioning of a system is dependent upon the quantity and quality of its input, output, and feedback.*

Input. Input into a system is the contribution of information, materials, or energy into the system. Input may come from one of the components or from outside the system. An open system receives a great deal of input, whereas a relatively closed system is receptive to very little input. The more open the system, the more varied and extensive is its input. All human systems are open systems.

The previously mentioned study of the care of surgical patients would be ineffective without extensive input. This input would be in the form of information, which would include, among other items, a description of procedures and techniques currently in use in each hospital, an analysis of the degree to which nurses and patients are conforming with established procedures and policies, and statistics regarding the incidence and type of postoperative infections during a given period of time. Conversely, input related to the heating system of a small house would be much more limited, since it is a relatively closed system.

Output. Output from a system is the end result of the processes of that system, and may be in the form of information, materials, or energy. Output from the digestive system would be in the form of waste materials, sources of energy, and information related to sensations of hunger or satisfaction. Output from the study of the system for caring for surgical patients would be information such as statistics and recommendations.

Feedback. Feedback is that portion of the output of a system that, when fed back into the system, enables that system to regulate itself.

Feedback enables the system to compare what *is* with what was expected or needed. If a person who is very hungry eats a single lettuce leaf, feedback from his digestive system will indicate that the lettuce leaf is not adequate to relieve his hunger.

Since feedback is a portion of the output of a system, it may be in the form of information, material, or energy. The information may be verbal or nonverbal. If a restless, uncomfortable patient falls asleep during a back rub, that behavior is feedback that enables the nurse to conclude that the back rub was effective. During range-of-motion exercises, resistance coupled with verbal or nonverbal indications of pain serves as feedback that enables the nurse to decide that the exercise should be discontinued until further evaluation of the joint has been made. Careful examination of vomitus, fecal matter, blood, and urine will give the nurse and physician feedback related to the functioning of various body systems.

Strictly speaking, feedback describes the status or condition of the system at a given point in time. In many systems, it does not indicate whether the condition is good or bad, better or worse. It does give the nurse data with which to make a decision or judgment. For example, a thermometer might indicate that a patient's body temperature is 101° F. That feedback, that information by itself, cannot indicate the action to be taken. If the nurse were in the process of sponging the patient because of a previous temperature of 103.8 ° F, the feedback of a body temperature of 101° F would indicate that the fever sponge bath had been effective and would be reassuring rather than a cause for concern. If, however, the patient were three days postoperative, had been running a normal temperature, and suddenly complained of a chill, the same feedback of a body temperature of 101° F would give the nurse reason to suspect that something was wrong with one or more of the patient's physiological systems, and that some type of intervention was needed.

Feedback comes from a component that has been affected by some action of the system, and is usually fed back to the component that initiated the action. It makes a circle or loop, commonly referred to as a feedback loop. One portion of this loop consists of output from one component (usually the one that was affected by the system) and the other portion becomes input back to the component that produced the effect.

It is important that the system receive feedback if it is to regulate itself, to grow more effective and/or efficient. For example, on a surgical unit, comments and complaints about a new type of dressing tray must actually reach the surgical procedure committee in order for the committee to learn that they made a poor choice of trays and to be able to make another selection. Output in the form of muttering and sputtering that is never directed to the appropriate component of the system does not become feedback. It remains output and is of little value.

The nurse consistently tries to get feedback from the patient, family, or community about the effectiveness of her nursing interventions. Since it is only through adequate feedback that a system can regulate itself, the nurse-patient interaction can correct itself, grow, and develop only when both patient and nurse obtain enough feedback to evaluate the system at frequent intervals.

SYSTEMS THEORY AND PATIENT TEACHING

Three specific systems that are of concern to the nurse are the patient, the family, and the community. The patient is a complete system, composed of many subsystems or components such as the circulatory and nervous systems. The patient in turn is a component of the family system. Every family, whether it be large or small, nuclear or extended, traditional or nontraditional, functions as a system that is capable of interacting with the nurse and other components of the health care delivery system. The family is a component of the community system, which may include other members of an isolated commune, other families in an apartment building, the neighborhood, a small town, or even a city.

The Patient

In some acute care settings, such as the recovery room or an intensive care unit, the nurse must focus almost exclusively upon the patient. The various systems of his body are threatened and urgent physiological needs must be met. In some situations a psychiatric nurse will interact with a single patient for an extended period of time. In each situation the nurse is well aware that the patient is a component of a larger system of family and friends, but for the moment, top priority for nursing intervention belongs to the individual patient system.

The Family

In nonacute settings, and during visiting hours in acute care settings, the nurse extends the boundaries of the patient care system to include persons who are significant to the patient. Since interactions within the family system influence the patient's response to illness, therapy, and recovery, the nurse makes every effort to include the family when explanations are given, decisions are made, teaching is done, and feelings are explored.

Failure to include the family may negate the effectiveness of patient teaching. For example, extensive teaching and planning with a newly diagnosed male diabetic, the dietician, and the nurse may prove futile in the long run if the wife who has always prepared his meals is not included.

The need for family involvement is quite obvious in some situations, but in others the need is more covert. For instance, a married woman who has had a mastectomy may apparently do well in the hospital environment. As a patient, a single system, she may seem to function well and adapt effectively. Upon discharge, however, she ceases to be an individual patient system and again becomes a component of the family system. Her mastectomy has affected her, and whatever affects her must of necessity affect her family in one way or another. Any teaching that focused entirely upon the patient must be deemed incomplete and is likely to prove ineffective. If she was not taught to cope with family feelings, questions, and concerns, whether expressed or not, she may of necessity resort to interactions that are not conducive to either family unity or good health.

Sometimes the nurse's interaction with the family system may be secondary to her interaction with one member of the family. At other times the nurse's primary intervention is with the family as a whole. A community health nurse may help a family prepare to receive a premature baby, an infant with birth defects, or an adult from a nearby psychiatric hospital. The nurse may never have seen the individual about whom the family is concerned; her priority is the family system, of whom the individual will soon be a significant component.

The Community

The nurse, especially a community health nurse, often interacts with the community as a system. This may occur for one of two reasons. First, an individual patient or family may be the primary focus of the nurse's teaching but, because of the nature of the problem, the boundaries of the system must be set beyond the family to include all or part of the community. It may be that special transportation is needed for a handicapped schoolchild, volunteers may be needed in a crisis-ridden household, funds may be needed from the local Shriners organization to help a severely burned child, or education may be needed to overcome resistance of a small group of neighbors to the return of a young man from a drug detoxification facility. In each instance, effective nursing interaction recognizes the patient and family as a component of the community system. The nurse may not be the one who actually interacts with the relevant segment of the community, but it is her assessment of the situation, and her knowledge of systems theory, that facilitates the appropriate action.

The second reason for a nurse's interaction with the community as a system is that she may be called upon to teach a segment of the community. She may be asked to teach first aid to a group of cub scouts, to teach high school students about venereal disease, to promote better sanitation at a migrant camp, or to discuss the effects of stress with businessmen on a televised talk show. In each instance, the nurse will study the system and obtain input from the involved persons to determine what the group needs and wants.

Each of the groups to be taught is a small system that interacts with other systems within the larger system of the community. Since whatever happens to one system affects the other systems to some degree, it is impossible to *effectively* teach one group without affecting a number of other groups. Only with a bland, easily forgotten presentation or program is the effect likely to be confined to the original system. (In effect, *nothing happened* to that system.) A program on venereal disease, for instance, that is effective for high school students will affect, in one way or another, the parents, younger brothers and sisters, the local newspaper, the school board, local church groups, and many others. Some of these effects will be desirable, and some will be undesirable, but the nurse who is knowledgeable about systems theory will anticipate these interactions between the component parts of the community system.

Working with Systems Theory

Once the nurse has identified the system with which she will be working (patient, family, or community), it is important to identify or acknowledge the boundaries of that system. These boundaries may be physical, temporal, psychological, functional, and so on. The physical and temporal boundaries for a nursing student might be the unit of an assigned patient, from 7 to 11 A.M. Four persons might be included in the system in the functional roles of student, patient, instructor, and team leader. Each of these four people will function both as a separate system and as a component of the larger patient care system. Anything that happens to one of these four persons during the morning will affect the other three to a greater or lesser degree. Each one is receiving input from many sources into his or her own system, which in turn influences that person's input into the larger system.

Input from the patient into the system might be his reaction to pain and discomfort, his anger over his poor prognosis, and his anticipation of relaxation following a bath and back rub. Input from the student is likely to be her enthusiasm for nursing, her eagerness to please the patient, her instructor, and the team leader, and her apprehension and anxiety over her ability to cope with the patient's pain and anger. The team leader's input is her insistence that all assignments be completed on time and her concern for a beloved patient who is dying in the next room, while the instructor's input is support and assistance for the student.

Additional input from other sources intrudes upon this system and affects the relationships within it. A late or cold breakfast tray, the unexpected arrival of the patient's priest, the frowns of a group of doctors making rounds, or the death of the patient next door—any such input will affect one or more of the component persons directly and the others indirectly.

A working knowledge of systems theory enables the nurse to identify many of the various inputs into a given system and to anticipate the possible effects upon the component parts as well as upon the system as a whole. The nurse's knowledge of herself as a system enables her to recognize the variety of forces that are acting upon her and to acknowledge possible ways in which her responses to this input may influence her input into the patient care system.

4

Maslow's Hierarchy of Needs and Patient Teaching

Abraham Maslow, a distinguished psychologist who died in 1970, felt that the best way to understand human motivation was to study the most highly developed, fully human persons he could find, persons who were exceptionally productive, healthy, creative, happy, and mature. He studied the lives of hundreds of persons ranging from presidents and artists to homemakers and scientists. Despite their many differences, these people had one thing in common; they were all described by Maslow as being self-actualized.

Maslow concluded from his research that human beings are dominated by a number of basic needs that tend to direct a person's behavior until each need is satisfied. Although these basic needs are interrelated, they tend to be hierarchical in nature. The lower-level needs must be satisfied before higher-level needs can be met. In fact, the higher-level needs do not even emerge until lower-level needs have been satisfied, at least minimally. For example, a man's need for food can at times dominate his behavior. His mind will be preoccupied with thoughts of food, any available physical energy is likely to be expended upon attempts to get food, and he may even behave in a dangerous and irrational manner. Once his need for food has been met, and his hunger has been relieved, higher needs will emerge, and these higher needs will then dominate the person until they are satisfied.

Maslow identified the following needs as being basic to human motivation: physiological needs, safety and security, love and belongingness, self-esteem, and self-actualization. Of these needs, man's physiologic needs are the most basic, the most powerful, and the most obvious. These needs include his need for oxygen, liquid, food, shelter, sleep, and sex. If one or more of these needs is not met at least minimally, the person will be unable to meet higher-level needs. A

25

person who is suffocating from lack of oxygen may also have unmet self-esteem or security needs, but they will be ignored until he is no longer panicky about his oxygen supply, and until he is able to breathe adequately with minimal effort and exertion.

As soon as physiological needs have been adequately met, a group of needs that Maslow describes as safety needs emerge. These needs include both physical and psychological safety and security. When both the physiological and safety needs have been met, the belonging-ness and love needs emerge, followed in turn by esteem and self-actualization needs. The need to know and to understand, and esthetic needs, are among the highest-level needs.

Although the basic needs usually emerge in an order similar to the one described above, they do not form an absolute hierarchy. There are many exceptions. The potential for satisfying higher-level needs may be dulled in persons who have lived at a bare subsistence level for many years. A psychopathic personality may be unable to give and receive love even though his lower-level physiological and safety needs have been adequately met. Some outstanding persons have devoted their lives to ideas or causes with almost complete disregard for their own basic needs. Maslow believed that persons who have been born into situations that enabled them to satisfy their basic needs very early in life develop such strong unified characters that they can withstand the loss or frustration of these needs for considerable lengths of time.

Most people manage to satisfy many or most of their lower-level needs, but from time to time a few of these needs may be unmet or only partially satisfied. During an illness or in time of crisis, a person may experience a sudden upsurge of unmet lower-level needs. It is these unmet needs that have the greatest effect on a person's behavior and that most significantly affect the nurse-patient interaction. Once a need has been satisfied, it has little effect on behavior and motivation, since a need that has been met is no longer a need.

Maslow's hierarchy of needs provides a useful theoretical basis for assessing the patient or client's condition, anticipating needs, planning nursing intervention, and understanding the patient's response or lack of response to nursing intervention, including patient teaching.

There are two essential steps in using Maslow's theory of basic needs as one of the bases for patient teaching. First, you must be able to recognize the signs, symptoms, and behaviors that might indicate an unmet need. Second, you must be able to determine how the unmet need might affect the teaching-learning process. In the pages that follow, I will describe some of the indicators of unmet basic needs and will describe some of the effects on patient teaching.

PHYSIOLOGICAL NEEDS

Oxygen

Inability to meet the need for oxygen results in the most urgent of all emergencies. All tissues are susceptible to lack of oxygen, but the brain is permanently damaged within a very few minutes by inadequate oxygenation. Emergency resuscitation measures may restore respiration, and the patient may recover, either partially or fully, from the episode. During this time there is no doubt that a basic need is not being met. In other situations, however, the patient's condition is less dramatic, and the unmet need for oxygen may be unnoticed or overlooked.

Indicators of an Unmet Need for Oxygen. Information related to the need for oxygen is obtained from your assessment of the patient's pulse, respiration, color, alertness, and composure. A pulse that is difficult to palpate, labored or difficult respirations, pallor or cyanosis of the skin, mental confusion, lack of energy, or apprehension may indicate an unmet need for oxygen.

Implications for Teaching. Since a person's physiological needs must be met before higher-level needs can emerge, his need for oxygen must be met before patient teaching can be effective. Before starting to teach, you will need to make a quick assessment of the patient's oxygenation and take any action that may be indicated. If the patient is in any sort of respiratory distress, attention to his psychological status will be an integral part of meeting his physiological need. Fear, anxiety, or apprehension can increase a person's need for oxygen and at the same time make respirations more ineffective, more difficult, or more labored.

In addition to improving the patient's psychological status, you can help the patient by attending to those factors that facilitate effective oxygenation. Elevation of the head of the bed and the use of extra pillows may ease the discomfort of orthopnea and enable the patient to concentrate on learning. A person with respiratory disease may be exceptionally susceptible to impure or polluted air. He must be protected from people who smoke and be assured of adequate ventilation in his room. If the patient's breathing is dependent upon one or more pieces of equipment, you will need to check the functioning of the ventilator, the patency of the tracheostomy tube, or the adequacy of any other equipment before you attempt to teach. It may be necessary to reposition the patient in order to facilitate optimal chest expansion and respiration. In short, you must assess the situation and do whatever is necessary to help the patient meet his need for oxygen if he is to be able to attend to his higher-level needs, including the need to know.

Fluids

The impact of prolonged or extreme thirst and dehydration upon higher-level needs is quite obvious. No one would attempt to interest the dehydrated survivor of a boating accident in discussing art or politics; his need for fluids is overwhelming. The more common deprivations of liquid are less obvious and can be overlooked. Varying degrees of dehydration may be found in persons with diarrhea and/or vomiting who are not under medical or nursing supervision, and in persons who are not fully mobile and therefore may not be able to obtain liquids at will.

Indicators of an Unmet Need for Fluids.   A careful assessment of the patient's condition may reveal one or more of the following: poor turgor of the skin, dryness of the mouth, lips, skin, and hair, constipation, and dark-colored urine with a higher-than-normal specific gravity. Since fluid and electrolyte imbalance are so interrelated, the patient may also exhibit some degree of mental confusion, irritability, or sluggishness.

Implications for Teaching.   Although the patient may not complain of discomfort or thirst, the stress of an unmet need for fluid may cause both physical and psychological discomfort, and the person who "does not feel very well" is often unable to concentrate upon learning. In addition, a dry or cracked tongue and lips may make it uncomfortable for the patient to speak and hard for him to interact with you as you teach.

If you discover that the patient's fluid intake is inadequate, the next step is to determine the cause. The patient may be unaware of the need for more fluid, and he may cooperate fully if he is taught how much he needs to drink each day. A patient may not be drinking simply because he is unable to reach the fluids easily, perhaps because of the pain of arthritis or the limitations of a stroke. Dislike of the fluids offered may be the cause. A child may refuse water or juice, but may eagerly drink

Kool-aid or eat popsicles. The advantages of adequate fluids may outweigh the negative aspects of cola and other soft drinks for an adolescent. If the patient is not drinking because of nausea or difficulty in swallowing, parenteral fluids may be necessary.

Although it may take a number of days (or even longer) to restore an adequate fluid balance, teaching will be more effective if the patient's need for fluids is met at least minimally.

Food

Except in situations involving famine or disaster, you are unlikely to encounter a starving patient. You will, however, frequently need to intervene in situations in which the patient and his family are malnourished or undernourished. Once you suspect that a person's nutrition is inadequate, all your skill in assessment and diagnosis must be used, because the psychological, social, cultural, and physical aspects of nutrition make it one of the most complex of the basic needs.

Indicators of Unmet Need for Food. Some of the clues to unmet food needs are: unplanned weight loss, failure to grow or gain weight, pallid skin, dull hair, listlessness, and lack of energy. Rather than assuming that these symptoms or conditions are caused by disease, you should consider, in the initial assessment of the patient, the quantity and quality of food eaten. Although none of these conditions, taken singly, would necessarily indicate interference with higher-level needs, when taken collectively they could indicate that the person may be functioning at a level so minimal that there is little energy for, or interest in, learning and growth.

The indicators listed above are often the result of the inadequate food intake of an undernourished person. Similar effects may result from an adequate intake of poor-quality food (malnourishment).

If the basic need for food is equated with optimal nutrition, then excessive weight gain and obesity may be considered indicators of an unmet basic need.

Implications for Teaching. Adequate nutrition is essential for physical fitness, a sense of well-being, and the energy needed to meet high-level needs. Therefore, the malnourished or undernourished patient cannot be expected to have much energy available for learning. In some situations, the person's nutrition must be improved before extensive or long-range teaching can be effective. In other situations, teaching is needed before the person's nutrition will improve. A careful nursing diagnosis is needed to differentiate between the two types of situations.

An elderly widow, living alone, may be undernourished and losing weight because: a) she can't afford enough food, b) she may be too feeble to prepare three meals each day, c) she may have no appetite because of illness or loneliness, or d) she may have no way of obtaining groceries regularly. A nurse who "scolds" the lady for not eating, or "teaches" her about the need for adequate nutrition, will accomplish nothing. The lady's self-esteem is lowered by the scolding, and the basic situation remains unchanged.

Unmet nutritional needs cannot always be equated with un-availability of food. Fad diets, preference for junk foods, irregular patterns of eating, ignorance, or psychological quirks can contribute to poor nutrition. Parental neglect and child abuse, illness, pride that forces one to reject food stamps or welfare, and psychological problems can also block satisfaction of the need for food.

Since many of the factors that influence a person's food intake have emotional overtones, a gentle and accepting attitude on your part helps the person to explore the problems related to his unmet nutritional needs. Once a nursing diagnosis has been made, you can then initiate the necessary teaching. You may need to contact other appropriate members of the health care team, or a community group such as Meals on Wheels, for help in solving the problem.

Shelter

Although very few persons in this country are without shelter, many millions live in substandard or hazardous houses. Shelter from ex-tremes of heat and cold is necessary for life and is therefore one of the lower-level needs in Maslow's hierarchy of needs. Except in an emergency or disaster, the basic need may be not for shelter as such but for maintenance of a normal body temperature, as in the case of the patient with extensive burns. Rapid changes or prolonged extremes of environmental temperature are especially difficult for very young, elderly, feeble, or inactive persons, and an abnormal body temperature is stressful to all people.

Indicators of an Unmet Need for Shelter or Maintenance of Normal Body Temperature.   Some of these indicators are: color and condition of the skin, body temperature, position of body, and level of activity and alertness.

Some physiological responses to extremes of heat and cold are dramatic and obvious, such as burns, frostbite, sunstroke, shivering, and sweating. Other responses are less intense but equally significant indicators. Such responses to cold include sluggishness, a huddled-up posture, a curled-up position in bed, rubbing one's hands, pulling one's clothes around the body more snugly, and lower levels of energy and attention. Responses to heat include restlessness, irritability, loosening one's clothes, thirst, lethargy, and decreased attention span.

In most instances the response to an extreme of temperature does not vary with the cause. The body's response is the same whether the extreme of temperature is caused by disaster, neglect, or therapy. The body's response to cold, for example, is the same, with variations in degree, whether the cold is caused by a blizzard, an unheated house, a hypothermia machine, or extreme airconditioning, and the effect of the unmet need for warmth on higher-level needs is the same.

Implications for Teaching. It may take a very careful assessment and a great deal of perception to discover that a patient's apparent lack of motivation, attention, and general unresponsiveness is due to the discomfort of being too warm or too cold. Either condition detracts from one's ability to meet higher-level needs and interferes with the teaching-learning process. Neither shivering nor sweating is conducive to learning. Since changes in body temperature take place slowly, you may need to delay your teaching until the patient's body has responded to whatever nursing measures are taken to make him comfortable. It may take days for an elevated temperature to subside; it may be an hour or so before a chilled patient feels the full effect of extra blankets or sweaters and a hot drink.

Sleep

Each person's need for sleep must be adequately met on a fairly regular basis if he is to function at an optimal level. Satisfaction of the need for sleep is dependent upon both the quantity and quality of sleep and is affected by the person's diurnal rhythm. When normal patterns and rhythms of sleep are interrupted by illness, insomnia, work, or the environment, the resulting fatigue and stress limit the probability of meeting higher-level needs.

Indicators of an Unmet Need for Sleep. Some of these indicators are rather obvious, such as dark circles under one's eyes and falling asleep during the day. Other signs include a lowered level of energy and motivation, irritability, difficulty in concentration, slowed reactions, and lowered mental acuity. Since some of these indicators are symptoms of illness, you will need to validate your assessment in order to determine whether the behaviors you have observed are the result of illness or of inadequate sleep.

Implications for Teaching.   Whenever possible, teaching of the patient who is tired and tense from lack of sleep should be delayed until he is more rested and alert. Fatigue makes learning much more difficult. If the lack of sleep is due to insomina, you may need to teach the patient how to slow down at the end of the day, and to develop a soothing ritual of activities prior to bedtime that is conducive to sleep. If a person's schedule simply does not allow enough time for adequate sleep, you may need to help him evaluate his priorities and his lifestyle as you encourage him to meet his basic need for sleep. In any event, you will not try to teach him when he is tired or sleepy.

Sex

Maslow includes sex as one of the basic needs that must be satisfied in order for the higher-level needs to be met. Although sexual behavior is influenced by many needs, especially by the love and belonging needs, Maslow stresses that love and sex are not synonymous, and states that sex may be studied as a basic physiological need.

Because of the cultural, moral, and psychological aspects of sex, this need is perhaps the most difficult of the lower-level needs for the health care worker to deal with, especially when helping a physically handicapped, elderly, retarded, or institutionalized person. However, with the increasing acceptance of sex and sexuality as integral aspects of human life, the public will be expecting knowledgeable and concerned assistance in dealing with various physiological problems such as infertility, birth control, venereal disease, and menopause. In addition to the physiological aspects of sex, you may find it necessary to assist families with problems of sexuality that relate to their love and belonging, esteem, and self-actualization needs.

Indicators of unmet needs related to sex.   These unmet needs might be indicated by the following: difficult or painful intercourse, failure to conceive, painful menstruation, unwanted pregnancy, difficult or disturbing menopause, overt or excessive masturbation, and improper sexual advances.

Implications for teaching. In order to treat the patient as a whole person, you must be prepared to include sexuality in the assessment phase of nursing process, and to respond to any clues that might indicate that the patient has unmet needs related to sex. This will require a knowledge of human sexuality, the ability to facilitate open communication with a patient or client, and an awareness of your own feelings and attitudes toward sex.

Many nurses find it no more stressful to take a sexual history and to discuss the patient's sexual needs with him than to discuss his nutritional needs. Other nurses, because of their own culture, upbringing, and value system, find it difficult to do more than answer a patient's questions accurately and factually.

You may find that you need to spend considerable time and energy working through your own beliefs and value system. For example, if you believe that premarital sexual intercourse is a sin, you are likely to find it difficult to work as a public health nurse in a neighborhood in which many girls are sexually active at age 13 or 14, and where the rates of teenage pregnancy and venereal disease are high. Despite any personal difficulty, however, your interactions may be very effective if you recognize that you cannot and should not impose your values on other people. You need not approve of the behaviors you encounter in patients, but in order to function effectively, you must be able to accept each patient as a worthy and valued individual. A nonjudgmental attitude, regardless of your personal beliefs, will enable you to help your patients learn.

SAFETY NEEDS

Once a person's physiological needs have been met, the safety needs emerge. Up until this time, he may have had to take chances with his own safety in order to meet his basic physiological needs. When they have been adequately satisfied, he then begins to seek a safe, orderly, predictable world.

Although Maslow usually referred to safety needs as a singular need, there are two components to safety within the context of the health care delivery system: psychological and physical safety.

Psychological Safety

In order to feel safe and secure, a person needs at least a minimal understanding of what to expect in terms of people, interpersonal relationships, his bodily functions, routines, procedures, equipment, and other aspects of his environment. In most instances, the nurse can integrate the explanations or demonstrations that will meet the patient's safety needs with other activities during her early contacts with the patient. Some of these explanations will be based upon the nurse's ability to anticipate frequently encountered fears and anxieties, while other explanations are based upon the patient's comments, questions, and other verbal or nonverbal cues.

Indicators of unmet needs for psychological safety. These needs are difficult to assess because the related behaviors are easily misinterpreted. The person who fails to keep clinic appointments because he is awed and frightened by the clinic setting may be thought to be lacking in motivation. The patient who refuses the fluids that have been ordered because he is afraid of asking for the urinal too often may be labeled "uncooperative." The patient in a research center or teaching center who will follow only those orders issued by his attending physician or a familiar nurse because he is terrified of being "experimented on" is more likely to be considered obstinate than assessed as frightened. Much of the behavior that is labeled as uncooperative, difficult, noncompliant, or demanding does not stem from malice or ill-will on the part of the patient, but rather from his unmet safety needs.

An assessment of psychological safety needs requires considerable skill and patience. Since there is no readily identifiable set of indicators, clues must be sought in such diverse behaviors as frequent and often repetitious questions, unusually passive compliance or refusal to comply without extensive explanations, frequent or seemingly unreasonable requests, demands for a ritualized schedule or rigid routine, and the physiological signs of fear or anxiety.

Implications for teaching. Much of the early teaching in any setting is planned to relieve the patient's anxiety and help him feel comfortable. Once the initial explanations have been given, however, the focus of the teaching may shift rather rapidly from helping the patient to adapt to a new situation to an emphasis on "things he needs to know." If this shift is abrupt, or occurs too quickly, the patient's ongoing need for psychological safety will not be met and he will be unable to meet his higher-level needs. Unless a situation is relatively stable and unchanging, the patient's needs will change frequently, perhaps from day to day. Preoperative threats to safety and security will be replaced by postoperative threats, which may be followed in turn by apprehension related to discharge and the worries that often accompany convalescence. Since a worried, anxious patient is unable to concentrate upon things to be learned, the only teaching that is effective under these conditions is that which is designed to reduce anxiety and thereby facilitate future learning. An ongoing assessment of the need for psychological safety is critical throughout the patient-nurse interaction, whether it be in an acute care setting, clinic, or the patient's home. Failure to meet the psychological safety needs can seriously impede a patient's progress, whereas adequately met safety needs free the person to move to a higher level of need fulfillment.

Physical Safety

According to Maslow, safety needs do not emerge until physiological needs have been met. Although this is true for the patient, you cannot wait to attend to safety needs until physiological needs have been met. You will need to meet safety and physiological needs simultaneously. Since many safety needs cannot be identified by the patient or family who are not aware of the potential threats or dangers, the staff in the health care delivery system must assume almost total responsibility for meeting many of the physical safety needs.

Indicators of unmet physical safety needs. In some situations, there may be no indicators from the patient that a physical safety need was not met until his body responds to a threat or responds to injury. Examples of such bodily responses include: nausea from an incorrect or excessive dose of drug, joint contractures from poor positioning, muscle atrophy from inadequate exercise, fever from a nosocomial infection, bedsores from prolonged pressure over a bony prominence, and a bruise or fracture from falling out of bed. All of these are the result of an unmet safety needs. In terms of patient safety, it matters little whether the patient's body is responding to the effects of an act of commission or an act of omission by the nurse.

The patient's concern with physical safety is most frequently related to pain or discomfort, and may be indicated by a question such as, "Will it hurt?" Less direct expressions of concern may be missed or misunderstood unless the nurse responds to the tone and underlying feeling rather than the words themselves. Questions and comments such as the following more often indicate a safety need than intellectual curiosity: "How fast is my IV supposed to run?" "What makes that clicking noise in the machine?" and "I usually get a large and a small white pill in the morning. It's new to get two small ones."

Implications for teaching.   The patient and family need to be taught the possible dangers specific to a given age (such as accidental poisoning of toddlers), a specific situation (such as anticoagulant therapy) or a specific environment (such as highly waxed floors in the home of an aged person). They need to be taught how to protect themselves and others from injury, infection, and disease. They also need to be taught basic first aid, including mouth-to-mouth resuscitation, and the Heimlich maneuver for the person who is choking. The patient needs to be taught how to protect himself from complications related to his present disease or condition. Although the need for patient teaching related to physical safety needs may seem less urgent and less obvious than some other teaching needs, failure to do such teaching may seriously hamper or endanger the patient's progress.

Belongingness and Love Needs

When the physiological and safety needs of a person have been met, the need for love, affection, and belonging emerges. Each person yearns for affectionate relationships with people, and seeks a place for himself within each group in which he finds himself. If he feels relatively safe and secure, he will expend considerable energy to meet this need. Maslow differentiates between these love needs and sex, which he feels is a physiological need. His view of love closely parallels that of Carl Rogers, who has defined love as "being deeply understood and deeply accepted."

Maslow found that growth and the development of one's potential are inhibited by the absence of love. Clinicians have proven that babies who are not loved will fail to thrive, sicken, and may eventually die.

Within the health care delivery system, the need for love, understanding, and acceptance is often expressed as a protest against the frequent dehumanization of health care. These expressions of need range from the complaints of individual patients to documentary films about the inhumanity of some nursing homes. The patient or family member may comment that "Nobody cares, nobody knows how I really feel; I'm just another number in this hospital"; "If you dare to complain, it gets worse"; or "I've been waiting out here for three hours now—I don't think anyone even knows I'm here." Such feelings affect the patient's reaction to therapy, his response to teaching, and his motivation for recovery.

Indication of unmet love and belonging needs.   In accordance with the flight-or-fight responses to stress, the person with unmet love and belonging needs may either passively accept the situation or may actively seek to be noticed and recognized within the health care delivery system. Unless you are meticulous in your assessment of the patient or family, these responses may be misinterpreted, with little if anything done to meet the underlying need. The quiet patient who is feeling hurt and dehumanized may be described as a good patient and left alone, while the assertive patient who is also feeling hurt is described as a difficult patient and also left alone. In each instance the basic need continues to be unmet.

Assessment of the quiet, noncomplaining person is difficult. His behavior is not disruptive and may even be satisfying to the staff. He may seek approval and acceptance by being eager to please, agreeable, compliant, and easily satisfied. He may try to be helpful in order to feel that he belongs. Since all these behaviors may be misinterpreted or pass unnoticed, you will need to be especially thorough in your assessment of any patient who seems to be almost too good or too quiet or too cooperative.

Assessment of the person who is actively seeking a place in the unit or group is less difficult. The indicators of his unmet love and belonging needs may include frequent ringing of his bell, complaining about many things, both important and trivial, stopping by the nurse's station a number of times each shift, asking many questions, spending considerable time in the patient's lounge or the hall, and other types of attention-seeking behavior. Some of these behaviors tend to alienate the staff, and as they withdraw from him, his needs are unmet to an even greater degree.

Implications for teaching.   Satisfaction of love and belonging need starts with the very first contact with patient and family, and may precede other types of interaction. For example, in a clinic setting, prior to the appointment, eye contact and a smile in passing acknowledge the patient as a person. When you introduce yourself, and call the patient by name, you acknowledge him as a person and a member of the unit.

Teaching, which is based upon systems theory, acknowledges the interrelatedness of patient, family, and staff. The nurse recognizes the importance of the patient's ties to family and friends, and incorporates these relationships into her teaching. She avoids any action that would tend to widen the distance between patient and family, and actually structures her teaching to strengthen ties by including members of the family system whenever possible. She knows that teaching is likely to be more effective if it is mutually acceptable to members of the family system.

In addition to teaching the patient and family or friends how to grow and develop in their relationships despite the patient's condition or prognosis, you can do many things within an agency setting to meet the patient's love and belonging needs. In general, any nursing action that decreases the feeling of being ignored will help to meet the person's need for acceptance and belonging. In teaching situations, such fundamental behaviors as fully facing the patient, maintaining eye contact, and sitting down with him for a time whenever possible help him feel that you are reaching out to him in an accepting way. Mutual goal setting assures the patient and family that they are members of the health team, that they are accepted, and that they are understood. When a nurse plans the teaching with little or no input from the patient, she increases his sense of isolation and aloneness and reinforces his feeling that he does not count for much within the health care delivery system.

ESTEEM NEEDS

Although the esteem needs are sometimes treated as a single need, Maslow identified two sets of esteem needs. The first is self-esteem and self-respect, and the other is the respect and esteem of other people.

Self-Esteem

The esteem needs are critical for the promotion of health, especially mental health, even though health care workers sometimes place a much higher priority on physiological and safety needs. If the promotion of health is accepted as a goal of nursing practice, attention to the esteem needs must be as carefully planned and as deliberate as the attention to lower-level needs.

The self-esteem needs include the need for competence, skill, mastery, independence, and confidence. Although all persons do not enter the clinic or hospital with the same or even similar degrees of self-esteem and self-respect, it is important that each person retain his self-esteem, and that he leave with the same or greater degree of esteem and respect.

Indicators of unmet needs for self-esteem and self-respect. Unmet self-esteem needs are indicated by feelings of dependence, lack of confidence, lack of competence, and lack of ability. These feelings are likely to be reflected in statements such as "I just can't get around anymore, I guess I'll have to give up my job"; "Somebody will have to irrigate my colostomy for me—I just can't"; or "I'll never be able to stick to that diet."

Each person has his own way of dealing with unmet esteem needs. A few people will reveal their feelings, but many more will conceal them as best they can. All of your psychosocial assessment skills will be needed to differentiate between the quietly self-confident person and the person who, though outwardly assured, feels inwardly incompetent or inferior. As you make this assessment, it is essential to determine which aspects of any unmet self-esteem needs are part of a longstanding pattern of behavioral responses, and which ones are health-related or illness-induced. A successful lawyer who feels confident and respected in a courtroom may feel awkward, awed, and incompetent when confronted with braces, traction, a urinal, or an authoritarian physician or nurse.

Implications for teaching. The focus of patient teaching is directed toward the patient's acquisition of skills and understandings that will result in increased self-esteem and self-respect. This increased self-esteem may be noted in statements such as: "I *can* get around—today I got on and off the toilet alone"; "I'm learning to be an accountant so I can keep on working"; "I did it, and I never thought I'd be able to"; "I guess I really can take care of her at home"; and "I did it all by myself this time!"

The effort to maintain and hopefully increase the patient's level of self-esteem and self-respect must start with the first patient contact. Some of the initial patient teaching should help the patient to feel competent and to feel that he has retained a fair amount of his independence and autonomy. If the patient does not know how to do what is expected of him, he will feel awkward, helpless, or incompetent. Early patient teaching must make certain that the patient is able to fill out his menu, call for the nurse, and get to the bathroom (or use the bedpan or urinal). It is vital that the patient be *able* to do these things, rather than merely *know how* to do them. The person who has been told what to do, but is unable to do it because of arthritis, confusion, pain, anxiety, or some other reason, will suffer from an increasing loss of self-esteem.

Respect from Others

In addition to feeling good about one's self, a person needs to know that others share that feeling and opinion. Maslow believed that a stable and healthy self-respect is closely related to *deserved* respect from others. This need for respect and approval of others can be noted in patient questions such as, "How am I doing, doctor?" and "Am I doing it right, nurse?" The person who is trying to stop smoking, to calculate a diabetic diet, or to walk with an artificial leg needs feedback and reinforcement. Each needs to know that people whom he considers important feel that he is becoming more capable and more competent in the areas with which he has been struggling.

Indicators of unmet need for respect from others. These indicators may include the following: decreased motivation, minimal expenditure of energy, and discouragement. A person, consciously or unconsciously, usually tries to live up the expectations of those who are significant in his life. If other people seem to be disinterested, or seem unimpressed by his efforts, he may well figure, "Why bother? I'm not getting anywhere." If others seem to expect him to fail, he is likely to do so. On the other hand, if you are interested and aware of the patient's progress, a genuinely enthusiastic "You're doing fine" or "That's better than you did yesterday" will tend to raise the person's self-esteem and spur him on to even greater effort.

Implications for teaching. It is not enough to teach the patient *how* to do those things that he is expected to be able to do with respect to his health care. Teaching must include giving encouragement and positive reinforcement as the patient progresses, and acknowledging with empathy and support the inevitable periods of discouragement and frustration.

HIGHER-LEVEL NEEDS

Maslow defined the basic needs described in the preceding pages as deficiency needs, because each one meets the following conditions, among others:

1. Its absence breeds illness.
2. Its presence prevents illness.
3. Its restoration cures illness.

As a result of his later research, Maslow discovered another list of needs in still higher categories, which he calls growth needs, as opposed to the basic deficiency needs. All of these higher needs, which include the need for self-actualization and esthetic needs, are related to the delivery of health care, but their application is beyond the scope of this book. Maslow states that "living at the higher need level means greater biological efficiency, greater longevity, less disease, better sleep, appetite, etc. The psychosomatic researchers prove again and again that anxiety, fear, lack of love, domination, etc. tend to encourage undesirable physical as well as undesirable psychological responses. Higher need gratifications have survival value and growth value as well" (34, p. 98).

5

The Patient's Need and Right to Know

The patient and his family need and have the right to acquire the knowledge and skills that will enable them to function at an optimal level despite the limitations or restrictions of their current situation. The knowledge that is needed may be divided into three areas: 1) knowledge of the patient's physicial and/or mental condition, 2) knowledge of the health care delivery system, and 3) knowledge of the patient's immediate environment. The skills that must be acquired are those that will enable the patient and the family to feel competent and to attain at least minimal control over the outcome of the present situation.

KNOWLEDGE OF PATIENT'S CONDITION

In general, the patient and his family have the right to know as much as desired about the patient's condition. Although the amount of material presented and the manner of presentation will depend upon the age, ability, interest, and condition of the patient and family, the information must at all times be accurate, honest, and understandable.

Patients differ in their search for knowledge, partly because of their individual reactions to health and illness, and partly because of their personal concern or lack of concern for details. The person who never reads the details of a lease, contract, or guarantee may show little concern for the details of a Consent for Treatment form. The person who habitually responds to difficulty or trouble with "I don't want to hear about it" may react in similar manner to information related to his diagnosis, treatment, and prognosis. Other persons find considerable comfort and security through the acquisition of knowledge.

With respect to the patient's condition, there are at least six major areas of concern about which most patients seek information and about which they should be knowledgeable. These areas are: 1) language and terminology, 2) anatomy and physiology, 3) diagnosis, 4) prognosis, 5) therapy, and 6) predictable events.

Language and Terminology

Just as you needed to learn the appropriate medical terms in order to communicate with the physician and to understand professional litera-ture, so the patient needs to understand the words and abbreviations that are relevant to his situation. This knowledge is necessary for effective communication and for adequate understanding of sub-sequent teaching. In addition, it can be demoralizing for the patient to feel that he is the only person who does not understand or comprehend what is being said.

Anatomy and Physiology

The patient can participate more fully in his own treatment regimen, whether it is preventive or therapeutic, if he is knowledgeable about his body and its functioning. You may assume that the patient and his family understand basic anatomical and physiological concepts, but many people are woefully ignorant about their own bodies. Sometimes this lack of understanding is apparent from even a casual interaction, such as the announcement by a patient in the waiting room of an orthopedic surgeon that she needed to have an operation to "fix the cartridge in my knee." It was evident that the woman knew little or nothing about the structure of her knee in general, or about cartilage in particular.

One of the difficult tasks of teaching is to assess how much the patient already knows, and to determine the minimal knowledge that is necessary for adequate understanding and cooperation on the part of the patient. The concept of minimal knowledge is important, because it is so easy to overwhelm a patient with far more information that he needs or is able to use. Basic information, presented in an atmosphere conducive to learning, frees the patient to seek additional knowledge as desired.

Among other things, the patient needs to know the normal values for relevant measurements and laboratory tests, as well as the norm for his own condition, in order to understand, and to some extent interpret, changes in his own condition. For example, he needs to know both the range of normal blood pressures and his own pattern of readings in order to understand the significance of a specific blood pressure.

Diagnosis

Except under unusual circumstances, the patient needs to know the nature of his illness or condition. If a diagnosis has not yet been made, he needs to know the name and purpose of the diagnostic tests, and the outcomes or results as soon as they are available. It is usually the prerogative of the physician to give this information, but you can support and encourage the patient to seek the information he needs if his physician does not volunteer it.

An uncertain diagnosis is anxiety-producing. Your role is to minimize the patient's stress as much as possible by telling him when, where, how, and by whom the tests will be done, why the test is being done, and what he will experience during the test.

Prognosis

Once the diagnosis has been made, the patient needs to know what it will mean to him, what the outcome is liable to be, and what is likely to happen to him in the days that lie ahead. You may need to help him put his concerns into words so that he can discuss them with his doctor. An open, honest, and frank discussion will relieve the patient of unwarranted worry and will enable him to make realistic plans for the future. He and his family need an opportunity to explore the impact of the patient's condition upon the family system. In some situations, extensive teaching may be needed by one or more members of the family before they can accept the patient back into the system, especially when the patient's prognosis necessitates extensive or difficult adjustments within the family relationships.

Therapy

The patient and his family need to know: 1) that they have the right to accept or reject treatment that is offered, 2) what the alternatives or other options are, 3) what the outcomes might be, both with and without treatment, 4) that a second opinion may be desirable (and that it will be paid for by some insurance plans), and 5) the meaning of informed consent.

Before the patient and physician or nurse agree upon a treatment regimen, the patient needs to know the anticipated or hoped-for results, the nature or any risk, side effects, or adverse reactions, and the cost in terms of time, energy, money, and discomfort. The patient needs to know the name and dose of any drugs that are prescribed, as well as possible side effects and incompatability with other drugs, alcohol, or foods.

Predictable Events

One of your greatest contributions is your ability to provide anticipatory guidance. "Forewarned is forearmed" is as true in the area of patient teaching as in any other aspect of life. The patient who knows what to expect is better prepared to cope with a given situation than the patient who is taken by surprise by fairly common events or happenings. For example, the young mother who learns that her difficulties with her two-year-old child are common to the "terrible two's" stage may cease to worry that she is a poor mother or that her child will continue to be a source of frustration.

One patient may need to know in advance the nature and probable duration of discomfort after surgery. Another may need to know that pospartum "blues" are common, to be expected, and not abnormal. You can help a family understand some of the predictable responses to the home dialysis of one of its members, and help a spouse to anticipate the changes in behavior that accompany the various stages of dying.

The process of teaching about predictable events varies from patient to patient. Some patients are future-oriented and are able to read about or discuss events that may not happen for a number of weeks or months. Other patients learn best at a time closer to the event. They are not as concerned about what *will* happen as they are with what is happening *now*. In either case, your task is to help the patient and family explore and cope with situations that, although understandable and predictable, are unique and unknown to this particular patient and family.

KNOWLEDGE OF THE HEALTH CARE DELIVERY SYSTEM

The question "Have you ever been hospitalized before?" is asked of almost every patient. The answer is duly recorded but is rarely used as part of the data base for patient teaching. This is extremely unfortunate, because effective health care is dependent to a large extent upon the patient's ability to function within that part of the health care delivery system that is relevant to him, whether it be a clinic, the Visiting Nurse Association, or a large medical center.

The patient's need for knowledge of the health care delivery system is related to his need for psychological safety, his need to belong, and his need for self-esteem. You can help satisfy these needs by teaching the patient those things that will help him feel confident of his ability to manage himself within a vast and often impersonal system. Your teaching should include material related to four areas that are of concern to the patient and his family. These areas are: 1) personnel, 2) organization and structure, 3) routines and procedures, and 4) norms and expectations.

Personnel

First of all, the patient needs to know the names of the persons with whom he is directly involved. This seems almost too obvious to mention, but all too frequently the nurse or other health care worker fails to introduce herself, especially in a clinic or emergency room setting. Once the initial introduction has been made, the patient needs to know the role or position of the person, whether she is a staff nurse, head nurse, a "float" whom he will probably never see again, or his primary and permanent nurse.

The person who is entering a large teaching hospital for the first time needs to learn the difference between an intern, resident, and attending physician, as well as the difference between the medication nurse, the treatment nurse, and the floor nurse, and so on. In some situations it is important for the patient to have some sense of the hierarchy of the institution, and to learn the channels of communication, both official and nonofficial. In some institutions it is hard for patients to differentiate between the professional and nonprofessional staff, especially if many or all of them wear colored uniforms without caps.

Organization and Structure

The patient often needs to learn the relationship of one agency to another, or one department to another. He needs to know what resources are available within the agency or within the community and what the routes of access are. He needs to know that there are often a variety of options and alternatives from which to choose; for example, the person who must lose weight might seek help from Weight Watchers, an obesity clinic, a specialist, or Overeaters Anonymous.

You may need to interpret the role of a given member of the health team and clear up the patient's misconceptions before the patient is able or willing to use the service that is available. The patient may not accept the services of the medical social worker, for example, because of his belief that social workers are "for poor people who can't pay their bills."

Routines and Procedures

Upon occasion, the nurse may be the person who explains complexities of the health care system, interprets (or cuts through) the red tape and policies of the agency, and assures the patient that certain requirements are routine and not personal.

Norms and Expectations

You may need to help the patient learn what he can expect of the staff and what the staff expects of him. There will be less irritation, frustration, and misunderstanding, if expectations are open and discussed as needed. For example, a patient may feel angry or distraught because the clinic physician does not tell him the details of his condition and therapy. The physician's position may be, "I'll tell him anything he wants to know, but he never asks, so I assume he knows as much as he wants to." You may need to teach the patient in this situation that the physician expects each patient to seek the information he desires. Another common difficulty caused by differences in expectations arises when a patient in pain believes that "if they want me to have a shot, they'll give it to me," whereas the staff assumes that "if he needs something for pain, he'll ask for it."

Much knowledge about norms, expectations, and limits is gained through trial and error or by observation, but in many situations the patient can acquire the needed knowledge more quickly and effectively if you deliberately teach him those things that will enable him to participate effectively in his own care. This is especially true of children and adolescents, who tend to be more assertive in their search for norms and limits, and who may unintentionally irritate or alienate the staff in their efforts to discover what is expected of them and what they, in turn, can expect of the staff. Persons who are passive, shy, or unsure of themselves often need extra help in this area.

KNOWLEDGE OF THE IMMEDIATE ENVIRONMENT

The security and safety of the patient is closely related to his understanding of his current environment. He needs to know: 1) the nature of any real or potential hazards, 2) the name and location of things and places, and the time when various events will occur, and 3) the details of routines and procedures that involve him.

Hazards

Since patient safety is basic to all nursing interventions and to all aspects of health care, the patient and/or his family must be taught about any real or potential dangers or threats to safety. In the patient's home, you may notice peeling paint that might endanger a toddler, scatter rugs on a polished floor that might cause an older person to fall, or a too-soft mattress on the bed of a person with orthopedic problems. Inappropriate use of pillows coupled with inactivity can cause contractures, whereas excessive stress and pressure may endanger the mental health of a family.

In an acute care setting, the patient needs to learn what things might prove dangerous with regard to the use of oxygen, chest suction, or IV's. He needs to know how to help protect himself against infections, both from other people and from contaminated equipment. He needs to learn the essentials of medical asepsis, including such basic tenets as "Don't walk around the hospital unit barefooted," and "Don't use objects that have been on the floor."

People, Places, Things, and Events

The patient needs to know the name and role of persons who will be significant to him. He needs to know the location of the emergency exit, the telephone, the bathroom, and the storage space for his clothes. He may be unfamiliar with the objects named emesis basin, urinal, chux pad, commode, and so on. He needs to know the time and duration of visiting hours, when meals are served, and when he will be awakened. He may need to know the difference between the recovery room, the intensive care unit, and a progressive care unit.

Routines and Procedures

The patient needs to know such things as when and how he will receive any bills or charges, that he will, in a teaching hospital, be cared for by a number of doctors, that the anesthetist will visit the night before surgery, and whether or not the agency assumes any responsibility for personal belongings. In one situation, a patient needed to know that shifts changed at eleven PM and that the nursing staff were busy at that time, because she had concluded that "they all go for coffee about eleven—so you might as well not ring for anything then."

In short, the patient needs to know enough about his environment to feel relatively safe and comfortable.

SKILLS

In addition to knowledge about his condition, the health care delivery system, and his immediate environment, the patient needs to learn a number of skills in order to feel competent and maintain his self-esteem. He needs to be able to do both those things that are expected of him and those things that he either wants to do or feels compelled to do. These skills include such diverse abilities as being able to read a thermometer, change a dressing, incorporate a special diet into family meal planning, bathe a newborn baby, walk on crutches, and so on. In addition, he needs to know how to participate in his own care and how to help himself. In order to do this, he needs to know how to recognize and report changes in his condition or situation, how to interact effectively with both his family and professional persons, how to make appointments with a clinic or an unfamiliar health care center, and how to cope with regulations and frustrations. He also needs to learn to apply basic decision-making skills to his options as a consumer of health care.

6

Teaching and Nursing Process

Nursing process can be described as a systematic way to organize the activities of professional nursing into an effective framework for nursing practice. Nursing process is an orderly sequence of steps or phases that enable the nurse to combine the most relevant elements of the scientific method with the most desirable elements of the art of nursing. The use of the scientific method alone could produce technical, competent, but dehumanized patient care. Reliance upon the art of nursing alone could give warm, gentle, empathic nursing care that is likely to be haphazard and often ineffective. The use of nursing process enables the nurse to combine knowledge with intuition, art with science, warmth and spontaneity with deliberative action.

THE PHASES OF NURSING PROCESS

There are many descriptions and definitions of nursing process, and different authorities use different terms to identify its various steps and aspects. For the purpose of this book, nursing process will be described in terms of five phases: assessment, diagnosis, planning, intervention, and evaluation. Each of these phases will be discussed briefly, and then the relationship between nursing process and patient teaching will be described. (See the bibliography for more information on nursing process.)

Assessment

The assessment phase of nursing process might well be called the foundation or keystone phase, for the total process can only be as effective as its assessment phase. During this phase the nurse engages in activities that have been described in various terms, such as collecting data, sizing up the situation, obtaining a data base, or analyzing the system. In the simplest terms, the nurse obtains the necessary information about the patient or client from a wide variety of sources. These sources of information include: a) people (the patient, family, other nurses, doctors, aides and orderlies, other members of the health team, members of the clergy, visitors, neighbors, and so on), b) physical findings, (such as physical signs, height, weight, biopsies, lab work, X-rays), and c) records and reference materials (patient's chart, textbooks, professional journals, films and slides, and the like).

During the assessment phase the nurse processes the information she receives: she sorts, categorizes, verifies, questions, analyzes, retains, and discards various portions of it. Since some information is neither useful nor important, you need to be able to select the information that is relevant to your situation. This may change from hour to hour or day to day. The nurse in the recovery room may not find it useful to know that the parents of the six-year-old patient with an emergency appendectomy are in the process of obtaining a divorce, but the nurse on the pediatric unit may find that information most helpful in understanding the child's behavior during visiting hours.

Diagnosis

Once the nurse has selected useful and necessary information from a variety of sources, a nursing diagnosis can be made. This diagnosis will indicate the status or condition of the patient or client in terms of his responses to real or potential threats to his mental or physical well-being. This diagnosis is made in a manner similar to a medical diagnosis, in which the physician takes the relevant facts, organizes them, and arrives at a diagnosis. This may be a tentative diagnosis if additional information is needed.

A medical diagnosis usually indicates a disease or condition, stated in terms that have been classified and accepted by the medical profession. This classification system facilitates communication between physicians. A system for categorizing and classifying nursing diagnoses is being developed that will enable nurses to communicate more effectively about nursing care.

A medical diagnosis usually states or refers to a specific disease, while a nursing diagnosis is more closely related to human responses to conditions such as pain, immobility, disturbances in elimination, anxiety, and the like. A nursing diagnosis represents a synthesis of input, an integration of information, into a concise description of the patient's current adaptation. Authorities differ as to whether or not a nursing diagnosis can indicate a healthy state or successful adaptation. A "healthy" nursing diagnosis would indicate that the patient or client was coping effectively, both mentally and physically, with his situation, disease, or condition. Some authorities feel that a nursing diagnosis should reflect a problem that is amenable to nursing intervention.

Many patients are likely to have more than one nursing diagnosis, just as they are likely to have more than one medical diagnosis. Multiple nursing diagnoses can sometimes be dealt with simultaneously (such as difficulty in ambulation and decreased appetite), while at other times it is either advisable or necessary to set priorities (a nursing diagnosis of difficult respiration conveys a greater urgency than a second diagnosis of limited range of motion). A nursing diagnosis provides a guide for nursing intervention. A change in diagnosis usually indicates the need for a modification or change in nursing actions.

Planning

Planning can be no better than the quality of assessment and the accuracy of diagnosis. If essential data were not collected, if critical facts are not known, if the nurse is unaware of some aspect of the situation, the assessment will be inadequate, the diagnosis will be inaccurate, and the subsequent planning ineffective.

During this phase the nurse selects from possible nursing actions those which she feels will best meet the needs of the patient. She will also decide at this time how and when these actions will be implemented. During this phase, the nurse establishes the outcome criteria for each of the planned actions. She decides how she will know if each action is effective: what she will observe and how the patient will respond. Outcome criteria are essential for the last phase of nursing process, evaluation. Unless the nurse knows the desired result of an action, she will find it difficult to evaluate that action.

Just as input from the patient was vital during the assessment phase, so it is during the planning phase. The nurse may need to make some initial decisions about possible courses of action, but in most instances the patient needs to be involved at some point in planning for his own care. He needs to help develop the goals and objectives, to select activities that are compatible with his value system and his life style, with his expectations and his available energy.

Intervention

Intervention, the fourth phase of nursing process, includes all those actions that are needed to implement the plans made in the preceding phase. Since the nurse set outcome criteria for each intervention, she is well aware of the result she is seeking, of the effect that is desired as the patient responds to the intervention. Since the nurse knows what she is trying to accomplish, and has determined how she will know whether or not she is successful, she is able to monitor her intervention and to modify her actions as she goes along in order to achieve the desired outcome.

Evaluation

Evaluation is the process by which the nurse systematically seeks to determine the effectiveness of her nursing care. She compares what actually happened with what she expected or hoped would happen. She examines the outcome of nursing care by measuring it against the criteria she had previously established during the planning phase.

One of the strengths of nursing process is that evaluation is not haphazard or left to chance. It is expected, deliberate, and planned in advance. It enables the nurse to improve the quality of care by determining which interventions were helpful and which were not and, in many instances, by discovering why interventions were or were not effective.

If the evaluation of nursing care indicates that the actual outcomes were not the same as the desired outcomes, the nurse proceeds to evaluate each phase of the process until the reason for less-than-optimal outcomes can be explained. An evaluation of the assessment phase will be based upon questions such as: Did I have all the necessary information? If not, what was missing? Was the information accurate? Current? Relevant? Any omissions or errors in the assessment phase will affect each of the other phases and influence the final outcome. This is because a faulty assessment leads to an incorrect or inappropriate diagnosis, which in turn causes poor planning, with subsequent ineffective nursing intervention.

Although a faulty assessment almost inevitably leads to ineffective nursing care, a *good* assessment does not automatically insure effective nursing care. It is possible to have all the necessary information and then interpret it incorrectly and reach an incorrect diagnosis.

A thorough assessment followed by an accurate nursing diagnosis is likely to facilitate an effective plan of care, but it does not guarantee this. If there is a wide range of possible nursing actions, the nurse might inadvertently choose a course of action that has only a minimal chance of being effective in the situation.

Finally, the nurse evaluates the actual intervention. A well-done assessment, diagnosis, and plan may fail to achieve the desired results because the nursing actions were unskilled, improperly carried out, or poorly implemented.

Evaluation enables the nurse to identify the reason for failure to reach the desired outcome. Evaluation makes it possible for the nurse to look for patterns of success or failure. If she finds, for example, that the majority of her difficulties are caused by a fuzzy or imprecise diagnosis, she will be able to improve the quality of her nursing care by seeking help in formulating precise nursing diagnoses.

NURSING PROCESS AND TEACHING

Patient teaching is a nursing intervention and, like any other nursing action, it is planned, implemented, and evaluated within the nursing process. Teaching is also a process, similar in many ways to nursing process. The teacher may describe her activities in terms of assessment, planning, intervention, and evaluation.

Assessment Phase of Teaching

The first step in teaching is the assessment of the learner, the teacher, and the teaching situation. Data must be collected about the learner's ability to learn, his physical and psychological readiness to learn, the medical and nursing diagnoses, his physical condition and prognosis, the treatment regime, his attitude and motivation. This information is needed so that you can accurately describe or diagnose the specific patient teaching situation.

Although a classification of teaching diagnoses has not been developed, it is possible for you to prepare a short statement that indicates the patient's needs related to teaching. Such a statement, usually in the form of a goal or objective, is based upon your assessment of the learner and will indicate the most important elements of the patient teaching situation.

Planning Phase of Teaching

As soon as adequate objectives have been developed, you can begin to plan what, how, when, and where you will teach the patient. Input from the patient that was obtained during the assessment phase will be used in making preliminary plans, which will then be discussed with the patient, usually before the plans are finalized. The patient's input is reflected in the goals and objectives that will direct the teaching. During this phase, outcome criteria are established that will enable you and the patient to evaluate the effectiveness of the patient teaching.

Intervention Phase of Teaching

This phase includes all the activities of teaching, such as demonstrating, explaining, reinforcing, testing, and rewarding. These activities will be described in detail in the section on methods of teaching.

Evaluation Phase of Teaching

This final phase enables you to determine the effectiveness of your teaching as measured in terms of the objectives and criteria. You can evaluate the patient's learning to date and, depending upon the outcome, make additional assessments and make provision for additional or remedial teaching, as needed.

SUMMARY

The phases of nursing process, when applied to patient teaching, provide the nurse with a systematic approach to a very complex activity. This deliberate and orderly process need not be cumbersome or slow. Once you become accustomed to using each of the phases in sequence, the teaching process will be equally as effective in a brief encounter in a clinic or in the patient's home as it is in teaching within a complex situation over a long period. The teacher who *seems* to teach by intuition, spontaneously and effectively, is a person who has mastered the phases of the teaching process, although she may not refer to them by specific names or labels.

AN ACADEMICALLY ORIENTED ALPHABET OF
PATIENT TEACHING

A is for Assessment   First step in the teaching-learning process
B is for Behavior   A change in behavior indicates learning
C is for Criteria   Contributes to both learning and evaluation
D is for Data   You cannot make an assessment without it
E is for Evaluation   Must be done at periodic intervals
F is for Family   Must be included if teaching is to be effective
G is for Guidance   Much teaching will be anticipatory guidance
H is for Health   The ultimate goal of nursing
I is for Information   A prerequisite for patient teaching
J is for Joint   It's the joint responsibility of patient and nurse

K is for Knowledge   A fundamental attribute of teaching
L is for Learner   A key person in the teaching-learning process
M is for Maslow   His hierarchy of needs cannot be ignored
N is for Nurse   The facilitator of patient learning
O is for Objectives   Difficult to develop but essential for planning
P is for Process   Teaching and learning are aspects of a process
Q is for Questions   The ability to formulate them is critical
R is for Readiness   Assess the patient's readiness to learn
S is for System   Input, output, feedback—all are important
T is for Teaching   An integral part of all nursing
U is for Understanding   The second level of Bloom's taxonomy
V is for Validation   The process of checking out one's perceptions
W is for Wisdom   A goal seldom fully achieved
X is for Unknown   There are many unknowns in education
Y is for Yearly   Make a yearly appraisal of your teaching skills
Z is for Zest   A necessary ingredient of patient teaching

THE REAL-WORLD ABC'S OF PATIENT TEACHING

A is for Advice — Don't give it (unless it's asked for)

B is for Backs and Back rubs — Opportune times for teaching

C is for Confusion — Who is teaching which patient what

D is for Doctors — Some help and some hinder

E is for Excuses — "Not enough time" for example

F is for Fidgeting — A cue that your teaching is off target

G is for Guarantees — There are none in patient teaching

H is for Helping — Helping toward health—your motto

I is for Initiative — You have to make the first move

J is for Jargon — Translate into plain English, please!

K is for Knowledge — If you don't have it, get it

L is for Listen — Above all, LISTEN!

M is for Mutual — Patient and nurse together, all the way

N is for Needs — Start where the learner is at—with his needs

O is for Obstacles — There are many

P is for Preaching — Don't!

Q is for Questioning — It takes a great deal of skill

R is for Relevance — An overworked term, but still important

S is for System — Remember the system

T is for Telling — What teaching is not

U is for Unpredictable — What the joys and rewards of teaching are

V is for Validate — Validate your data. Validate your hunches

W is for Wait — Talk less. Wait before you jump in with a reply

X is for Xerox — Each patient is different! There are no duplicates

Y is for You — Bearer of heavy loads, receiver of precious rewards

Z is for Zero — There is zero space left

PART II

THE TEACHING-LEARNING PROCESS

ASSESSMENT

7

Assessment of the Learner

As we noted in Chapter 6, the effectiveness of any nursing intervention depends upon the quality of the preceding assessment and diagnosis. The same is true in patient teaching. Effective teaching depends upon an accurate and complete assessment.

Assessment is not in any way specific to nursing or teaching. It is always the first step in any rational, deliberative activity. An extensive and comprehensive assessment is carried out before a Presidential trip abroad, the development and promotion of a new product, or the building of a new interstate highway. On a lesser scale, a chef would not agree to prepare a dinner party in a private home without making a careful assessment. He needs to determine the number of persons invited, the kind of utensils available, the type of fuel, size of the budget, the amount of counter and work space, the menu, and the expectations of the hostess. Even the routine activities of daily life require the same assessment process. One does not even plan the evening meal without checking the ingredients, time, and energy that are available.

DATA FOR ASSESSMENT

With respect to patient teaching, there are three major categories of data to be obtained: 1) data relevant to the patient's diagnosis, 2) data *about* the patient, and 3) data *from* the patient.

Data Related to the Nursing and Medical Diagnoses

This information provides the nurse with the knowledge needed for effective nursing intervention. It may be found in textbooks, professional journals, and hospital or agency protocol, as well as from other health care workers and former patients. From this material you are able to formulate your input into the teaching situation. The patient will make known what he needs and wants to learn, and you will know the content that should be included. The nurse and patient may identify identical, similar, or dissimilar content, but through a process of sharing and mutual agreement all critical areas will eventually be included.

Data relevant to the diagnosis would include answers to questions such as the following: What does the patient need to be able to do in order to live with this condition? Under what conditions should the patient seek further nursing or medical care? What problems have been encountered by other patients? What "helpful hints" might be effective? What kind of reactions are likely to be experienced by the family? What does the physician feel that his patient needs to know in order to cope with the condition or situation? Information relevant to the diagnosis enables the nurse to select general concepts that she can then apply to a specific patient situation. It enables her to assume responsibility for the overall focus and direction of patient teaching. Unless data relevant to the diagnosis are collected and used, the teaching is likely to be ineffective. A nurse could be warm, interested, supportive and yet lack the knowledge and information that the patient needs.

Data about the Patient

Objective data that describe the patient can be obtained from a wide variety of sources. Observation of the patient yields information related to sex, race, approximate age, general physical and mental condition, and overall capacity for sight, hearing, and speech. The patient's chart or referral form gives the highlights of his medical history, present condition, prognosis, and current therapy. The location and appearance of the patient's home gives some indication of socioeconomic status, and the records or chart may give family composition, occupation, birthplace, and religion. Information related to educational background or intelligence may be deduced from conversation with the patients, and occasionally from his choice of reading materials. I must emphasize that all data *must be verified with the patient*—otherwise you are operating on assumptions only. I remember one patient whose occupation was listed as toll-taker on an interstate highway. The books he was reading were ancient history and philosophy, and he indicated that he assumed his present job after a major heart attack a few years earlier. An impoverished senior citizen in a run-down inner city home may be a retired college professor who was educated abroad. Both his past experiences and his present situation will affect his readiness and ability to learn.

Data from Patient

Some of the material most relevant to patient teaching can be obtained or derived only from the patient. Factors that influence his attitude toward learning, his background and motivation, his interest and readiness to learn, his needs and abilities can be assessed only in conjunction with the patient himself.

The effectiveness of this assessment is directly related to the nurse's communication skills. Your ability to receive, interpret, and respond to verbal and nonverbal cues will largely determine the degree to which your assessment will be accurate and complete.

QUESTIONS

This type of assessment requires you to formulate questions which will elicit the greatest amount of significant information in the shortest time. The following paragraphs will describe the uses and characteristics of questions, and an example of a learning assessment will be described.

The Uses of Questions

If you were to list the reason for each of the questions asked of you and by you during the past few days, you would likely include many or most of the following reasons. Questions are asked to:

1. obtain information,
2. show interest in another person,
3. indicate that you are knowledgeable enough to discuss the subject,
4. test another person's knowledge, authority, interest, and the like,
5. get attention,
6. seek reassurance,
7. provoke, irritate, challenge,
8. help another person think through a problem,
9. give advice indirectly ("You *surely* aren't going to . . ., are you?") ("You don't want to . . ., do you?"),
10. and for a number of other reasons.

Categories of Questions

Questions can be divided into two categories, narrow and broad. The narrow questions include those for which there is a predictable, expected, or correct answer. Broad questions are those which call for brainstorming, exploring an issue or problem, and evaluating or examining an outcome.

Narrow questions are useful in two ways. First, a narrow question enables you to obtain specific information or to assess a person's factual knowledge. The person is asked to list, to state, to identify, or to describe something. "What are the symptoms of diabetic coma?" "What is the function of the pancreas?" "What are the names and dosages of the medications you are taking?" "What immunizations has your child had?" Another use of a narrow question is to test a person's understanding of material he has learned. "What is the difference between insulin shock and diabetic coma?" "Why should you not start to toilet train your child when you are moving or there is some other major change taking place?"

For all narrow questions, there is a right or wrong answer, an expected or appropriate answer. The information obtained is limited but useful, and in many instances a narrow question is necessary in order to focus the patient's attention on a very specific topic. The most limiting question is the one that requires only a yes or no answer. Such a question is useful and sometimes essential during an interview. "Do you know how to do a breast self-examination?" or "Have you had a chest X-ray in the past year?" In general, however, a yes-no question should be avoided. It takes almost as long to ask as a broader question that would elicit more useful information. Broad questions enable you to explore a person's ideas, to learn how he feels, and to better understand how he views his situation and his world.

One major category of broad questions asks the person to predict, to postulate, to hypothesize. "What do you think would happen if. . . .?" "What do you think accounts for the change in. . . .?" "Why do you think your physician. . . .?" These questions have no correct answers, so the patient is free to answer fully and freely IF you accept each answer as valid and important. If you really believe that the patient has a right to his own ideas and beliefs, you must accept each answer as worthy of discussion. If you are quick to indicate that the answer is based on faulty reasoning, the patient is likely to resort to answers such as "I don't know" or "I never thought about it" in order to avoid your implied criticism. If the patient's response to your question reveals a significant lack of understanding, or a gross misunderstanding, subsequent questions and discussion will help him come to a better understanding of the issue, without being told that he is wrong.

A second major category of broad questions includes those that ask for an opinion, judgment, or evaluation. "What do you think would be best for. . . .?" "What would be the most helpful in trying to. . . .?" "Which of these possibilities would be most useful in. . . .?" In responding to these questions, the patient must base his answer upon a set of standards or criteria, a value system, or his own beliefs. Since these factors influence his behavior and actions with respect to his health care and health practices, the responses to such questions often are extremely significant.

Asking Questions

The ability to formulate effective questions can be acquired. Teachers in an academic setting learn to write good test questions by writing and rewriting them until each question is concise and clear. It is more difficult to learn to formulate oral questions, because you usually have only one chance (it is very tedious to listen to a person rephrase each question). The following steps are often helpful in learning to ask effective questions.

1. Slow down and THINK *before* you ask a question.
2. Decide what it is you want to find out.
3. Mentally rehearse a few questions until you have a question in mind that is likely to obtain the information you seek.
4. Listen to your question and to the answer.
5. Compare the answer you receive with the type and amount of information you had hoped to obtain.
6. Decide why your question was effective, or why you had to ask additional questions to get the needed information.
7. Keep a log of your successes and failures for a while in order to identify successful techniques as well as problem areas.

This process is not easy, but if you do it several times each day, you will probably notice a significant change in your ability to obtain essential information quickly and unobtrusively, without seeming to pry or probe.

ASSESSING THE PATIENT'S NEED FOR TEACHING

One of the most effective ways to assess your patient's need for teaching is the structured interview, in which you use a predetermined set of questions to obtain the information you need. These questions may be written as notes to yourself, printed on a form, or memorized. The questions that follow are examples that may help you get started. You will eventually develop a set of questions that are relevant to your own situation and with which you feel comfortable.

Introduction and Overview of Patient Interview Guide

This guide was designed to help you gather the information that is necessary for planning nursing care, especially patient teaching. You will notice that each question is relatively broad. Since each one deals with an *area* of concern rather than a specific detail or fact, the questions can be used for any patient, in any setting. The format would be applicable for use in the patient's home, a clinic, or a hospital. With slight modifications in wording, the questions could be used with persons of all ages, from children and adolescents to senior citizens.

The interview guide is divided into three parts: the past (questions 1–5), the present (questions 6–14), and the future (questions 15–20). With some patients you may choose to conduct the interview at three different times, completing one section at each time. In other situations you may choose to complete the entire interview at one time. As you become skilled in assessing your patients, you can integrate your questions into your overall nursing interaction and may not need to set aside a specific time for this type of interview.

Each question was designed to help you assess a specific aspect of your patient's perceptions, strengths, and needs. As you ask each question, keep in mind its *intent or purpose*. This will help you to listen for relevant information rather than getting sidetracked by interesting but less significant details.

Although there are innumerable ways to phrase the content of the 20 questions in this guide, it is suggested that you memorize the wording of these or similar questions for your first interviews. If you do not have to think about the wording of your questions, you are free to ask the questions more naturally and thereby help your patient feel more at ease.

Conducting the Interview

You may feel strange or even apprehensive as you start your first interview. Some of you may find it easier to ask the questions while bathing the patient, doing range-of-motion or any other fairly lengthy procedure that does not require your entire attention. Others of you will find that you need to concentrate fully on the interview. If you will be doing only the interview, pull up a chair and make yourself comfortable *after* you have made certain that the patient is comfortable and that it is a convenient time for the interview. Explain to the patient the purpose of the interview and that you may be making a few notes so that you will be able to remember the information which will help you plan his nursing care and patient teaching.

As you proceed with the interview, listen for cues that indicate a need to pursue a topic (probably at a later date) or to drop it, at least temporarily. Watch for verbal and nonverbal cues that might indicate that the patient is tiring and that you should complete the interview at a later time.

If any question seems to merit further exploration, make a note of your concerns so that you can resume the discussion at a later time. In most situations it is advisable to keep going with the interview in order to complete this initial assessment UNLESS there seems to be a *critical* urgency and immediacy to the patient's concern. The patient interview is primarily a tool for assessment, not intervention. The information obtained provides the information that is essential for diagnosis, planning, and intervention. Therefore it is important to complete the initial interview so that the planned intervention will be effective, making provision for further exploration of any interview questions that seem to warrant it.

PATIENT INTERVIEW GUIDE AND RATIONALE FOR QUESTIONS

Questions related to the past

1. *Would you tell me a little about yourself, your family, your way of life?*

   This question is asked to elicit data relevant to the patient's developmental stage, self-esteem, work, hobbies, family composition, and so on. You will need to read between the lines to determine whether or not the patient feels that his life is satisfying and meaningful, and whether or not he feels worthy and respected. Resist the temptation to ask questions and pursue small details.

2. *What sorts of things do you do or try to do to keep healthy?*

   Listen for attitudes about health and the prevention of disease. Does the patient seem to actively pursue health, or is he passive? Do his answers indicate a sense of autonomy, or a sense of being powerless to control his own health?

3. *What things in your life seem to make it hard to keep healthy?*

   Ask this question to determine the patient's perceptions of stressors, such as the high cost of food, irregular time schedules of family, easy fatigue, inadequate recreation, and cultural conflicts within self regarding health. It is not possible to "cover" all factors, so accept the patient's remarks as valid assessments of his perceptions at this point in time.

4. *How do you usually react to being ill?*

   This question may reveal attitudes of fear, denial, "It's God's will," or an overly rational approach. It may give clues to other types of behavior, such as changing doctors at frequent intervals.

5. *How do you like other people to treat you when you are ill?*

   Ask this question to determine a possible approach to this patient as you plan and give nursing care. For example, does the patient indicate a preference for being left alone, a need to be "pampered," or a need to assume a dependent role?

Questions related to the present

6. *What were the symptoms of this problem or condition?*

   Answers to this question will indicate the patient's perception of any problems with the family system. Answers will also indicate the patient's awareness of his own body (were the symptoms rather advanced before he even noticed or acknowledged them?). Listen for choice of words, ability to express self, and possible embarrassment in talking about symptoms.

7. *What did you do when you noticed these symptoms?*

   This question may reveal attention to early symptoms, denial or rejection of illness, attitudes toward self-treatment versus medical care, and patterns of response of patient to stress (fight or flight response).

8. *Did anything seem to relieve these symptoms, even temporarily?*

   Ask this question for clues to faith or trust in drugs, prayer, home remedies, and the like.

9. *What do you know about your illness or condition?*

   Listen for accuracy and adequacy of knowledge, vocabulary, and understanding of medical terms. Also listen for patient's perception of whether or not doctors and nurses tend to give or withhold information.

10. *What have you been told about the treatment and/or tests that have been planned for you?*

    Rationale for this question is similar to that for question 9.

11. *What have you heard about the likely outcome of all this?*

    Note that this question does *not* ask what the *doctor* has said, but leaves the patient free to quote friends, the newspaper, the doctor, or any other source that seems significant to him. This question may elicit specific factual information and/or cues regarding attitudes of fear, optimism, resignation, desperation, or anxiety. This is one of the most important questions because of insights it may yield into patient behavior and motivation.

12. *Who or what has been your chief source of information?*

    (This question may have been answered, at least in part, as the patient responded to question 11.) An absence of medical sources may indicate poor communication with doctor and nurses. Sources such as neighbors or friends have implications for patient teaching. Questionable sources such as tabloid newspapers and television need to be accepted *without* comment at this time.

13. *What would you like to know more about?*

    This question is vital because it gives you a chance to find out where the patient 'is at'. The patient's answers indicate his priorities, and give a valid starting point for patient teaching.

14. *What, if anything, don't you understand as well as you'd like to?*

    This question may indicate whether or not the patient feels that he ought to understand the things that may have been explained to him, or whether he feels free to reveal his lack of understanding without fear of being considered dumb or inattentive.

Questions related to the future

15. *What do you think will be the hardest part of this situation, illness, or hospitalization?*

    The answer to this question will indicate some of the major stressors for the patient at this time. The answers will vary from time to time with the same patient throughout the course of a given illness, both as the situation changes and as the patient feels freer to express himself. These stressors may include pain, lack of privacy, loss of independence, financial insecurity, separation from spouse, family, or lover, fear of mutilation or disfigurement, embarrassment, and so on.

16. *Many aspects of your life will be disrupted, at least temporarily, by the doctor's treatment, or by hospital rules and routines. Which of these disruptions may be hard for you to deal with?*

    The answer to this question may be related to the previous answer or it may be very different. The patient may answer in terms of patterns of sleep, eating habits, sex, social activities, limited communication, and so on. The answers will help set priorities for nursing intervention that will foster appropriate adaptation by the patient to his stressors.

17. *What do you think may be the major effect of this illness or condition on your family and yourself?*

    Answer to this question may give cues to patient-family relationships, to the nature and extent of family concern, understanding, willingness and ability to be involved in the patient's situation. It may also indicate the patient's ability to project and plan for the future, and the degree to which his appraisal of his situation is realistic and/or appropriate.

18. *What could the doctor and nurses do that would be helpful?*

    Listen for factual, specific information plus cues related to the patient's expectations and perception of the role of medical and nursing personnel.

19. *What could other people do to help?*

    Listen for cues related to attitudes toward asking for and/or accepting help from others. Also for information related to wishes and desires regarding help from family, friends, agencies, and the like.

20. *What would you like to be able to do to help yourself get better or be more comfortable?*

    This question is likely to reveal information about the patient's personal goals and aspirations. The answer may indicate dissatisfaction (such as lack of self-discipline in adhering to prescribed treatment) or feeling of inadequacy. It may reveal things that the patient could probably do for himself if he had the necessary support, equipment, permission, or whatever. The patient's answer may indicate his attitudes toward the prognosis, his recovery, and reality.

PATTERNS AND STYLE OF LEARNING

In addition to assessing the characteristics and needs of the learner, it is important to explore the ways in which he learns best. Twelve of the many factors that affect learning seem especially relevant to patient teaching. Each of these factors will be discussed very briefly, followed by an example of the type of question you might ask to assess that area.

Collecting the Data

1. *Communication.*   Since patient teaching is based largely upon a verbal interaction between you and the patient, it is important to assess his ability and willingness to communicate with other people, both verbally and nonverbally.

> Questions to Patient
> Verbal Communication:
>> Would you describe yourself as quiet or talkative?
>> Are you any more comfortable talking to one or two people than you are talking in a group?
> Nonverbal Communication:
>> How likely are you to express your feelings through your behavior and facial expressions?

2. *Listening.*   The ability to listen carefully and attentively is necessary for effective learning. If you discover that certain conditions make listening difficult for your patient, you may be able to avoid or remedy those situations.

> Questions
> Which of the following conditions make listening difficult for you?
>> listening in a stressful situation
>> listening despite distractions of one sort or another
>> listening to a person in authority
>> listening when you have personal problems
>> listening when you know you must act upon what you are being told
> Which of the following, if any, have you said about yourself?
>> "I heard it, but it just didn't register."
>> "I heard it, but my mind went blank."

"I hear everything that goes on around me."
"I can just tune everything else out."

3. *Observation.* Since many of the things you will teach your patient will require attention to details, coupled with good observational skills in general, a careful assessment in this area will give you some indication of how direct you will need to be in helping your patient to notice the details that are relevant and critical to your teaching.

Questions

To what extent might you use the following phrases to describe yourself?
"I saw it, but I didn't think anything about it."
"I seldom notice little things like that."
Which of the following is sometimes difficult for you?
being observant in a stressful situation
noticing *small* changes
noticing little things that might be important

4. *Reading.* If your earlier assessment indicated that the patient is literate, you probably also learned what his reading level is. In order to fully use his ability to read, you need to know how he learns through reading.

Question

What helps you to understand and remember what you have read?

5. *Memory.* Some of your patients may be confronted with a number of things to be memorized, ranging from lists of acceptable foods to the names and dosages of current medications. For some people this is easy; for others it is well nigh impossible. A careful assessment will enable you to identify and assist the patient whose memory is faulty.

Questions

What kinds of things, if any, do you find it difficult to remember (names, dates, facts, things to do, and so on)?
When you do not trust your memory, how do you usually manage?

6. *Questioning.* People ask questions for many, many reasons. With respect to patient teaching, it is important for you to identify two types of questioning behaviors. First, the behavior of a patient who rarely asks questions, who seems not to be curious. Second, the behavior of a patient who asks questions but who seems willing to accept any kind of an answer, a patient who is unselective and accepts anything he is told. In either instance, you will not be able to depend

upon the person to ask for information that may be relevant and necessary for his understanding.

Questions

In general, would you describe yourself as skeptical or gullible?

Are you more likely to believe or to question what you read or hear?

Under what conditions are you likely to ask questions?

7. *Attention Span and Concentration.*   You will need to determine whether a given patient will learn best from a long, uninterrupted teaching session or from a series of short ones. In addition, it is important to identify those persons who need a quiet place, free from distractions in order to concentrate.

Question

To what degree is your ability to concentrate influenced by your surroundings, the presence of other people, noise, poor ventilation, and the like?

8. *Learning a Procedural or Manual Skill.*   Some people find satisfaction in working with their hands. Other people feel inept or awkward when required to learn a task that demands manual dexterity and coordination. An adequate assessment in this area will enable you to plan your teaching in accordance with the patient's needs.

Questions

How would you describe your *ability* to learn this skill?

How would you describe your *feelings* about learning this skill?

Under what circumstances might you say (or want to say) any of the following?

"Just *tell* me how to do it, you don't need to show me."

"Show me how to do it, then let me do it."

"Let me try to figure it out and do it by myself."

"Let me figure it out and then you help me do it."

How would you describe your reaction to using electrical equipment?

How would you describe your reaction to using mechanical devices or mechanical equipment?

How would you describe your manual dexterity at present?

How much practice do you usually need in order to master a new skill?

How do you react to instruction or supervision when learning or practicing a new skill?

Your assessment of the two following areas will make it possible for you to take into account those emotional reactions that might interfere with the patient's ability to learn.

9. *Reaction to New Situations*
   Questions
   How would you describe the ways in which you most commonly
   react to a new situation?
   What things have you found helpful in a new situation?
10. *Reaction to Anxiety or Stress*
    Questions
    In general, what kinds of situations are stressful for you?
    Given a choice, do you usually try to avoid or escape from a
    stressful situation, or do you try to work it through or "fight it
    out"?
    What are some of the ways in which you usually react to stress?
11. *Goal Setting.*   The setting of objectives and goals for patient
teaching requires input from the patient and family. For some persons
this is an unfamiliar process. Although they have from time to time
made plans based upon personal goals, the process may have been
largely unconscious.
   Your questioning in this area will serve two purposes. It will help
you learn how your patient may approach the process of setting
objectives related to patient teaching and health care. It will also bring
the process of goal setting to a conscious level for the patient and help
him gain new insights into the ways in which he sets and works toward
his goals.
   Questions
   What types of goals or objectives have you set for yourself in the
   past?
   In general, how would you describe your goals (ambitious, limited,
   realistic, or whatever)?
   What kinds of help and assistance do you find most useful when
   you are trying to reach a goal?
   Under what circumstances, if any, is it difficult for you to either
   ask for help, or accept help when it is offered?
   What do you usually do when your progress toward a goal is
   discouraging or unsatisfactory?
   In what ways do you decide how well you are doing, or what
   progress you are making?
   What kinds of rewards do you find most satisfying (praise, a
   feeling of accomplishment, a gift)?
   How would you describe your ability to tolerate frustration?
   How would you describe your ability to make plans for ac-
   complishing a given task?

How would you describe your ability to organize your resources (time, energy, money, people, and so on) in order to accomplish what you have planned?

12. *Application and Use of Learned Material.* This assessment may give you a few clues regarding the patient's tendency toward complying with or ignoring both your teaching and the prescribed nursing and medical regimens.

Questions

Once you understand something, to what extent do you usually try to apply it to situations in your everyday life?

Is your usual tendency to follow directions as they were given, or to modify the directions?

To what extent do you tend to do things the way they have usually been done?

Making the Assessment

The manner in which you assess the way your patient learns best will vary from patient to patient. You may choose to be very direct with the person who is highly motivated, who knows he has much to learn and is eager to get started. He is likely to respond with interest if you describe the need for this assessment and proceed to ask questions like those given above.

If the patient is uneasy, apprehensive, or reluctant to learn, you may choose to be less direct. You can deduce the answers to some questions from knowledge gained during previous interactions. You will need to ask some questions, but they can be integrated into other conversations so that they are less obvious.

You may not be able to collect the data you need when you first ask the questions because the person may be unable to answer until he has had time to think. Most of us seldom think about our patterns of learning, and a common response is, "I never really thought about it before—I'll have to think about it."

USING THE ASSESSMENT DATA

The information from this assessment, coupled with information from previous assessments, will enable you to work with your patient to develop objectives and plans for the teaching and learning that is needed. You will have a rational basis for making decisions related to the optimal time of day for teaching, whether the teaching should be integrated into other nursing care or done during a special time that is set aside, whether a separate quiet place should be sought or whether a familiar though noisy setting is preferable, and whether individual teaching is needed or a group approach would be feasible.

It is important to use the information you have collected. You and the patient have expended time and energy in making the assessments, and such an expenditure should be reflected in the teaching and learning that follows. If the information is not used, it need not have been collected. The patient will be frustrated to realize that the information he shared with you has no effect upon the way he is taught.

The following data related to three young college graduates with the same diagnosis will illustrate ways in which your assessments of a patient can provide clues to factors that will influence the teaching-learning process. Each summary or profile includes five or six bits of information that are likely to be significant. In each case, much additional information acquired during the process of assessment was discarded as being irrelevant to the particular situation.

As you read each learning profile, pause for a moment to consider the implications of each item and to think how that information might affect your teaching.

Marsha (age 26): Enjoys people, does not like to be alone, does not like to talk about self or condition, believes that disease is a punishment from God and that "there is nothing anyone can do about it." Does not enjoy reading, describes herself as "sort of scatterbrained," rarely asks questions, states that she is a show-me person who is a bit clumsy and feels she will need "lots of help."

Joan (age 24): Describes herself as "quiet and introspective," prefers to be alone and is upset by lack of privacy in hospital, talented with many skills and hobbies, never ill before. Has a horror of seeming inept (remembers pressuring father to teach her the basics of driving before she took driver education in school so that she wouldn't feel stupid). Strict vegetarian, avid reader, feels she can learn quickly "if you just bring me the directions."

Mike (27): Never seeks medical attention except for an emergency or if illness lasts over two weeks, refuses to take drugs except for an occasional aspirin. Describes himself as a morning person who does all his serious reading before 6 AM, when he goes to work. Energy and interest levels drop sharply after 4 PM. Has long attention span, prefers to stick with a task for several hours, is precise and attentive to details.

These examples will enable you to compare the relative usefulness of information obtained from specific assessments and the information that is more frequently obtained. For example, the knowledge that all three of these patients are college graduates, white, employed, middle class, Catholic, Republican, and unmarried provides little guidance or direction as you try to plan efficient, satisfying, and effective learning experiences for each.

8

Assessment of Readiness to Learn

The phrase *readiness to learn* sometimes seems to be nothing more than a cliché. Nearly every book and journal article on teaching and learning advises the teacher to take into account the student's readiness to learn. Little information is available, however, on ways to assess readiness to learn.

Sometimes, readiness to learn is closely related to ability. For example, reading readiness refers to prerequisite skills, such as the child's ability to distinguish one shape from another, to note similarities and differences within groups of objects and symbols, and to establish a pattern of left to right eye movements. Readiness to learn is sometimes equated with motivation and interest: "It's time for me to go back to college and finish my college education." "She's really ready for ballet lessons."

Much of the material written on readiness to learn refers to persons in an academic setting who are basically healthy. While there are significant similarities between readiness to learn in an academic setting and readiness to learn in the context of health education and patient teaching, there are major differences. The most notable of these are related to health and time.

Health affects readiness to learn because the patient and his family or both are often deeply concerned about fundamental issues such as pain, disability, disruption of personal or family life, or dying. In such situations, the factors that affect readiness to learn are different from those that operate when the learner is free from such discomfort and stress.

The constraints of time are different in patient teaching than they are in an academic setting, where there is likely to be teacher-learner contact over an extended period ranging from a semester to a full school year. Within the health care delivery system, readiness to learn is sometimes assessed in relation to long-range goals; more often than not, however, the nurse is concerned with the patient's readiness to learn *at the moment*, perhaps within the limits of a one-hour visit to his home, or within the limits of an eight-hour shift in an acute care setting. Since the nurse's contact with a given patient or family is likely to be limited, her assessment of the patient's readiness to learn must be brief, basic, concrete, specific, and useful.

In terms of the criteria just listed, the material that follows is a viable and practical guide for health care workers in assessing readiness at the beginning of each teaching-learning interaction.

READINESS AND LEARNING

Readiness to learn is the first factor in the learning equation:

$$\text{Readiness} + \text{Instruction} \longrightarrow \text{Learning}$$

I have defined readiness to learn as *the state or condition of being both willing and able to make use of instruction.* The degree of readiness to learn depends upon the degrees of willingness and ability; therefore, a high level of readiness presumes that the learner is eager and fully able to respond to instruction. On the other hand, if either willingness or ability is diminished, readiness to learn is also decreased.

It is important to distinguish instruction from teaching. Teaching includes, among other things, both the assessment of readiness and the activities of instruction. Instruction is only a part of teaching, and therefore is not equal to it. It may be helpful to consider readiness to learn as the patient's input into the teaching-learning process, and to consider the activities of instruction as your contribution to the specific teaching-learning interaction.

In most situations, an assessment of readiness is made before instruction, and is a separate activity. It may be done quickly during the first five or ten minutes of a home visit or during the early part of an eight-hour shift. The instruction that follows is influenced by the patient's readiness to learn, but the assessment of readiness to learn is *not* influenced by the instruction that will follow. The quality, nature, method, or scope of instruction does not affect the patient's initial readiness to learn, although the overall teaching process will naturally affect future levels of readiness.

Both readiness to learn and instruction are essential for learning. If either readiness or instruction is missing or deficient, there will be less than optimal learning. Although a high level of readiness may facilitate some learning even if instruction is missing or poor, excellent instruction will produce little or no learning within a person who is not ready to learn. On the other hand, a high level of readiness coupled with effective instruction will result in an exciting and satisfying level of learning.

FACTORS THAT INFLUENCE READINESS

Most discussions of readiness to learn include the factors of motivation, intellectual ability, and past learning or past experience. While these factors are relevant to patient teaching and health education, two additional factors are especially significant. These are comfort and energy. These two factors, coupled with a regrouping of traditionally accepted factors, give four factors to be assessed in determining readiness to learn within the context of health education and patient teaching.

Comfort

The term comfort includes both physical and psychological comfort and is closely related to Maslow's hierarchy of needs, as presented in Chapter 4. Basic physiological needs must be met in order for the patient to be physically comfortable, and his security needs must be met in order for him to begin to feel comfortable psychologically. These lower-level needs must be met before higher-level needs emerge, before he is ready to learn.

Physical comfort. Physical comfort implies the absence of conditions or symptoms that, if present, would make a person uncomfortable. Six of the most common sources of discomfort are: pain, nausea or dizziness, itching, fatigue or weakness, hunger or thirst, and the need to urinate or defecate. Since these conditions are not directly observable, you will need to base your assessment of comfort upon the patient's description of his condition. You may get some indication of possible discomforts from the patient's record or chart. For example, you may notice that he was nauseated earlier in the day.

You cannot assume that a recent nursing intervention has eliminated a discomfort, or that an absence of complaints indicates comfort. The fact that the patient has received medication for his pain does not guarantee that he is now free from pain. A patient with cystitis or diarrhea may have used the bedpan only a few minutes ago but still be unable to pay attention to any type of instruction because of a recurring need to defecate or void.

You will need to validate each and every observation, as well as each and every assumption or conclusion. Before beginning any instruction, you will need to ask such questions as, "Are you uncomfortable in any way?" or "Has your pain (or nausea or itching) subsided enough for us to proceed with the lesson we planned earlier today?" You might well verbalize the possibility of future discomfort with a statement such as, "I know that you need the bedpan at frequent intervals, so feel free to interrupt at any time if you need it."

Psychological comfort. Psychological comfort implies the absence of emotions that, if present in more than minimal amounts, would make a person uncomfortable. Six of the most common of these emotions are fear, anxiety, worry, grief, anger, and guilt. You may notice behaviors or nonverbal cues that would lead you to suspect the presence of one or more of these emotions, but they are not directly observable, and each perception or tentative assessment must be validated. You may need to say something such as, "We had planned to discuss your medications this afternoon, but you look worried to me, and it seems hard for you to lie still. Is this a bad time for you to try to learn about your drugs?" or, "You seem very upset, as if something has happened to make you angry. I wonder if we shouldn't discuss your feelings before we tackle the problem of learning to use the walker."

Any intense emotion will preclude the possibility of effective involvement in learning. Although great joy and happiness would not ordinarily seem related to psychological discomfort, the effect upon readiness to learn is similar. It is immaterial whether a stressor is pleasant or unpleasant—all that counts is the intensity of the demand upon the body for adaptation to the stressor. Intense joy and intense sorrow may produce almost identical nonspecific responses; the resultant stress may be intense and incompatible with learning for a period of time. We are accustomed to excusing a person in deep sorrow from a given task: "He's just not *up* to it." We should probably be equally ready to excuse a person who is experiencing great joy and perhaps learn to say, "He's just not *down* to it." It may be impossible for the person to heed an admonition to "come down to earth and pay attention."

One attribute of a skillful nurse is her ability to modify her planned intervention on the basis of new data. If you discover that your patient is uncomfortable, either physically or psychologically, your most appropriate intervention would be to relieve the discomfort before proceeding with the planned instruction. An uncomfortable person is not ready to learn.

Energy

Another factor that influences readiness to learn is the amount of energy currently available to the learner. Man's energy is finite; it is not unlimited. If large amounts of either physical or psychic energy are currently being expended, there may be none available for learning. The amount of energy available for learning is closely related to the patient's physical condition, his reaction to his stage of illness, the current number of stressors in his life, and the degree of situational or maturational crisis. A patient who is literally fighting for his life in a critical care unit has no energy for anything else. A person who is actively denying his illness has little energy for learning about it. A young women who has just become involved in divorce proceedings may have little energy at the moment for learning about hypertension. An elderly person who has just been moved from his home to an extended care facility is likely to have little energy in excess of what is needed for the adjustments to an entirely new life style. In some situations the amount of energy available for learning may increase rapidly, within a few days; in other situations it may take a few weeks or even months for a noticeable increase in energy to occur.

Other factors that affect a person's energy are his body rhythms. Some people have dramatic peaks of energy during each day in accordance with their diurnal rhythms. For those persons who feel most alive and vibrant in the early morning hours, it is likely to be frustrating and unsatisfying for all concerned to plan teaching sessions for the late afternoon. Just so, the person who "doesn't wake up until noon" cannot learn effectively during the early morning hours. Ironically, it is often assumed that all patients learn equally well during the morning, as this is a time when many nursing students are on duty and plan to do their teaching.

Some persons are concerned with their overall biorhythms. There are three rhythms—intellectual, physical, and sensitivity—which occur in cycles of 23, 28, and 33 days, respectively. These cycles can be plotted and charted, and are taken into account by some persons when planning any significant event or activity.

It is difficult to assess the amount of energy available at any given time. Many persons are not accustomed to consciously scheduling activities to correspond to periods of peak energy, and so they do not bring up the topic. You will probably need to take the initiative and seek the necessary data through direct questions, such as, "Would you describe yourself as a morning person or an evening person?" or, "When do you have the most energy?" Careful assessment of a variety of behaviors over a period of time may be needed to accurately determine the person's stage of illness and the resultant amount of energy available.

Motivation

According to Abraham Maslow, man is motivated by a hierarchy of needs, in which higher-level needs emerge as lower-level needs are met. As needs are met, their power to motivate subsides, and new needs emerge. A satisfied need has no power to motivate, but it permits a higher-level need to emerge, which, in turn, motivates the individual.

Maslow's theory of motivation forms the basis for much of this book and provides the rationale for many of the nurse's teaching interventions. It is usually possible to determine whether or not a person's physiological needs have been met, but the task becomes more difficult with higher-level needs, because they are usually interrelated. A single need may be manifest through multiple behaviors, and several needs may contribute to a single behavior.

Usually it is not possible to deduce a person's motivation from the behavior he exhibits as he proceeds to meet a given need. We can infer, for example, that a patient who is intent upon learning all he can about his condition, treatment, and prognosis is probably highly motivated. But we cannot determine the nature of his motivation, need, or desire merely by observing his behavior as a learner. In fact, the patient may be unaware of his own motivation, and even if he is aware of it, he may be unwilling to share it with you.

The patient may be motivated to learn by a need or desire to:

- know and understand
- get well
- please others, especially the professional staff
- be able to return to work
- retain the label of "good patient"
- manage own care
- be able to detect mistakes, to protect self
- enjoy a higher level of wellness
- avoid complications

- avoid criticism, advice, displeasure of others
- or any of a variety of other needs or desires.

The behaviors that result from each of the diverse motivations listed above may be identical; the patient may lean forward, ask questions, take notes, ask for a fuller explanation, seek you out, request books and pamphlets, and show any of a variety of other behaviors that might indicate motivation to learn. It is important that you resist the tendency to assume that you know *why* your patient wants to learn. In any group of eager learners, all exhibiting almost identical behaviors, there may be as many sources of motivation as there are learners.

If sources of motivation to learn were known, some of them might be considered inappropriate by persons committed to the prevention of illness and the promotion of health. A person is "supposed" to want to learn because he wants to improve his physical and mental well-being, not, for example, because he is afraid of being scolded by his physician, wife, or son for noncompliance. I believe, however, that any motivation to learn is valid, and that the teaching interventions of the nurse must focus, first of all, on helping the patient or family member learn whatever he is seeking to learn. Later on, you may want to consider helping him explore different ways of interacting with his physician, wife, or son, but only if this seems warranted on the basis of a careful assessment of his family system. It may not be wise to disrupt his current adaptation to those interpersonal relationships. The point is, a patient's motivation to learn is uniquely his, and should be respected as such. Any comments or inferences from you that he "ought" to have a different motivation to learn merely adds to his stress, alienates him from your efforts to help, and undermines the teaching-learning process.

I don't want to imply that motivations are permanent and unchanging, or that you have no influence in this area. As you interact with the patient, he will grow, develop, and gain new insights into himself and his relationships with those around him. As he examines and explores his behavior and responses, his needs and motivations will change. But these changes are the result of personal growth; they are not the result of being told, either directly or indirectly, "Your motivations are inappropriate—you ought to be learning for other reasons."

In the preceding chapter I emphasized the importance of "starting where the learner is at." His motivation to learn is part of "where he is at" and must be accepted as such. In most situations your *immediate* task is to help him learn; it is not to change the basis for his motivation.

Your goal is to assess the *level* of his motivation; it is not to assess the basis of his motivation.

If behaviors that reflect motivation to learn were placed on a continuum, they would probably range from an overall posture of eagerness down through lack of eagerness and apathy to rejection of any effort to teach. The absence of any discernible desire to learn is closely related to the patient's perception of his situation and his expectations for the future. If he presumes that his situation or condition cannot be improved, if his past experiences lead him to believe that no amount of energy and effort is likely to help, he is not likely to be motivated to learn and to participate in his own care. The possibility of attainment is an important aspect of motivation; people tend to strive for those things that are real possibilities for them. If a patient rejects your teaching, saying "I can never do it anyway" or "Nothing can help me," contact with other persons who have success-fully mastered a similar condition or disability may increase his perception of the possibility of attainment and consequently his motivation to learn.

Capability

The first three components of readiness to learn, namely comfort, energy, and motivation are assessed primarily on the basis of subjective data provided by the patient. One can hypothesize or deduce from the learner's behavior something about his levels of comfort, energy, and motivation, but each hypothesis must be validated by the learner himself. The fourth component, capability, is more amenable to objec-tive assessment. Many aspects of capability can be observed, tested, and measured.

Assessment of capability must be made concurrently with, or after, the formulation of objectives and identification of prerequisite skills. In other words, you cannot tell whether or not a person is capable of learning something until you know what capabilities are necessary, until you know what attributes and abilities are required. Only when you have determined what is required can you tell whether or not the person possesses the required attributes and abilities and is indeed capable of learning. The prerequisite capabilities include factors re-lated to physical ability, intellectual ability, knowledge, attitudes, and skill.

Factors related to capability are influenced or determined by heredity, age, maturation, stage of development, past learning, physical and mental health, and environment. Some limitations of capability can be alleviated or removed. Inability to read can be remedied by education, inadequate strength by exercise, and poor eyesight by eyeglasses. Other capabilities that depend upon maturation or development cannot be altered. An infant cannot be taught to walk until his muscular, skeletal, and nervous systems are sufficiently developed. A child cannot understand abstract concepts until his cognitive abilities are adequately developed.

Assessment of physical ability.   If the patient is to learn or acquire a psychomotor skill, four aspects of physical ability must be assessed.

1. Size. Are the patient's height and weight adequate with respect to the task and equipment involved? Can a short, frail spouse learn to care for a much heavier patient?
2. Strength. Does the patient have the strength to follow the prescribed regiment? Does the middle-aged secretary who gets virtually no exercise have the strength to manage crutches and a long leg cast, especially up and down a flight of stairs?
3. Coordination and dexterity. Can a patient with a pronounced tremor of his hands learn to measure liquid medication safely? Can a rapidly growing adolescent who describes himself as clumsy learn to help his father with home dialysis treatments?
4. Senses. Is the learner able to see, hear, smell, taste, and feel well enough to learn the designated task?

Assessment of intellectual ability.   There are at least five factors to be assessed in order to determine whether or not the learner possesses the intellectual ability needed for the competence he seeks.

1. Basic mathematical skills—to calculate dietary requirements, read a thermometer, and so on.
2. Reading skills—to read directions, instructions, and so on.
3. Verbal skills—to communicate with others who are involved in care of self or family, to express self.
4. Problem-solving skills—to be able to assess situations and know when and how to seek help and assistance.
5. Ability to comprehend and follow instructions—to insure safe, effective care at home.

Assessment of past learning and previous experience. The accomplishments and failures of the past are reflected in the learner's current level of knowledge, attitudes, and skills and provide a basis for the expected new learning.

Knowledge. Does the learner know the basic concepts and facts he needs in order to understand the new material? For example, does the learner have the basic understanding of the anatomy and physiology of his own body that he needs to comprehend your explanations? Does the person whom you are planning to teach to change a dressing have a knowledge of microorganisms adequate for understanding the terms clean, sterile, and contaminated? Does the rural patient know how to get around the city, from one clinic to another?

Attitude. A person's past experiences tend to either attract him toward a specified goal or turn him away from it. The person's attitudes and value system may exert powerful influences upon his readiness to learn. For example, it would be helpful to assess whether or not the patient with hypertension appreciates the importance of keeping his hypertension under control before you proceed to teach him about the prescribed regimen. It would be useful to regularly consider questions such as, "Does the mother whom I am teaching about immunizations even share my belief that children should be immunized?" as part of your assessment of the learner.

Skill. Some of the skills essential for current learning may have been acquired in the past. If so, you should avoid repetitious reteaching. If not, you will need to teach them before you proceed. For example, when helping a person prepare for the arrival of an aged, terminally ill parent, it is important to assess the person's current skill in bathing, lifting, and feeding a helpless person.

Once you have assessed the various aspects of capability, you will be able to determine if the learner is capable of learning the new material or acquiring the new skill. In some instances the objectives may need to be restated to accommodate some limitation of the learner's ability. In other situations, preliminary teaching, treatment, exercise, or other intervention is needed to overcome a limitation or deficit of the learner. In rare circumstances, you may find that the proposed objectives are completely unrealistic in light of the learner's capability, and that entirely different goals must be set. Difficult as this may be, it is better to discover the discrepancy between expectations and capability as the result of careful assessment than to discover it as a result of the learner's failure to reach the stated objectives.

Readiness to learn is difficult to assess because there are as yet no clear-cut or tested criteria; nonetheless, it is imperative that you make at least a tentative assessment upon which to plan your teaching. As you develop your own process o of assessment, it may be helpful to formulate questions that begin, "How will a person behave if he. . . ?" The concluding portion of each question will be specific to your assessment. For example, "How does a person act if he has boundless energy? if he has very little energy? if he is not interested in learning? if he believes his situation is hopeless and sees no reason to learn?" As you become proficient in describing the behaviors that indicate a given level of comfort, energy, motivation, and capability, you may be able to develop a continuum of behaviors that you can use to quickly and accurately assess readiness to learn. It will be difficult, but not impossible. A number of years ago it might have seemed inconceivable that one could assess a newborn infant and obtain a numerical score that would accurately describe the physical status of the infant, and yet the development of the APGAR scoring system made it possible.

Most assessments of readiness to learn must be done quickly if the nurse is to be able to do any teaching within the limits of a home visit, a clinic appointment, or an eight-hour shift in an acute care setting. Readiness must be assessed before each teaching interaction, because the status and condition of the patient or family may change rapidly, from one visit to another, from one shift to another. Some assessment data will remain valid from one teaching interaction to the next, while other data will change. The learner's capability will remain fairly constant and motivation may change very slowly, but his levels of comfort and available energy may change dramatically within a very brief period.

9

Assessment of the Teacher

It is important to periodically examine one's beliefs about the relationship of teaching to nursing. Do you view patient teaching as part of the care of every patient, or do you consider patient teaching as one of many possible nursing interventions, to be used in some situations and not in others? Do you consider patient teaching to be an option or the right of every patient? Do you believe that every nurse should teach or that patient teaching should be done by specially prepared nurses? The answers to these and other questions will help you clarify your beliefs about patient teaching and will influence the priority you assign to teaching.

ASSESSMENT OF YOURSELF AS A TEACHER

In addition to examining your beliefs about teaching, it is important to assess four factors: your energy, attitudes, knowledge, and skill.

Energy

At any given point in time you have a finite amount of energy, both physical and psychological. Many factors influence the amount of each that is available for the practice of nursing in general and patient teaching in particular. The amount of satisfaction you derive from your work, the activities and stresses of your personal life, any professional activities beyond the requirements of your job, the state of your health—all these affect the amount of energy available to you.

Given high priority, teaching is likely to be done even with minimal available energy. With a low priority for teaching and a low level of energy, however, you are likely to respond to only an urgent or dramatic need for teaching.

Attitudes

Your effectiveness as a teacher will be significantly influenced by your attitudes toward the patient and toward the subject matter. You may not be aware of the extent to which your feelings affect your teaching; therefore, an honest appraisal of your reactions should be an integral part of the teaching-learning process, especially in situations that seem difficult or stressful.

Feelings about the patient. If you like the patient you are to teach, find him interesting, are concerned about him and anxious to help him, then teaching him will probably be a satisfying experience for both of you. If, however, the patient has sometimes been "difficult," seemed rude, appeared demanding, or displayed inappropriate behavior, you may have a negative attitude toward him that may make it difficult for you to approach his teaching with enthusiasm and eagerness.

The ability to accept a person without necessarily approving of his behavior is a skill that you can develop, just as you can learn to cope with conditions that you fear or cannot accept, such as child abuse, alcoholism, or addiction. In the meantime, while you are developing this skill of acceptance, if your attitude seems to interfere with your ability to teach a given patient, you may need to openly admit it and request that the patient or family be assigned to another nurse. Many of my colleagues consider such an action to be the easy way out, a "cop out," but I feel that the patient is vulnerable and that it is his right to be taught by a nurse who can respond to him with at least minimal concern and empathy.

Feelings about the subject matter. You may have very positive feelings toward a given patient and still encounter difficulties in teaching him because of the nature of the content. Every nurse has some topics with which she is less comfortable, and some of these areas of discomfort are significant enough to interfere with effective teaching.

For example, you may have no difficulty in teaching a patient who has had a myocardial infarction the things he needs to know about the physiology of his heart and yet have trouble teaching him about the sexual aspects of his rehabilitation. You may have had no difficulty in teaching a family over the years about childhood diseases, immunizations, and toilet training and yet find yourself under great stress when that same family asks you about contraceptives for the 14-year-old who has become very active sexually.

Some nurses find it difficult to teach in situations involving such things as disfigurement, mental illness, mental retardation, unrelieved pain, the use of extraordinary means to extend life, and massive birth defects. It will be important for you to be able to recognize the basis or cause of any reluctance or problems in teaching, to be able to identify areas that are stressful to you, and to take appropriate action. Neither you nor the patient is benefited when you refuse to acknowledge that your strong feelings might create a block or barrier to patient teaching. Honesty and a willingness to examine your own feelings are basic to a helping relationship.

You can help yourself in a variety of ways. Additional study and increased knowledge may relieve your fears, apprehension, or misconceptions enough so that you are able to function with increasing effectiveness. Consultation and conferences with your colleagues and members of allied disciplines may give you enough support, practical suggestions, and additional resources for you to create a helpful teaching situation for the patient and family. You may want to seek professional counseling, possibly for just a short period, as an investment in your personal and professional future.

Knowledge

Patient teaching is influenced by the nurse's knowledge of relevant content. Whereas high knowledge does not guarantee that teaching will take place, it increases the probability. An intense commitment to patient teaching almost inevitably leads to increased knowledge, because the nurse actively seeks the information needed to teach each patient. This search for knowledge will intensify with each passing year as you strive to keep up with new developments in nursing, and it will be one basis for a lifelong commitment to continuing education.

Skill

In assessing your ability to teach, you will be concerned with two types of skill: 1) the set of abilities related to the particular condition or illness, and 2) the skills basic to teaching. Both are essential; you must be able *to teach* him how to do it. For example, the nurse who plans to teach a young couple how to care for their premature infant must first of all be skilled in the care of premature infants, and second, must be skilled in teaching nervous, apprehensive parents.

SUMMARY

The effectiveness of patient teaching depends largely upon what the nurse brings to the situation. Teaching is likely to be ineffective, or at best minimally effective, if one or more of the following are present: low priority, low energy, a negative attitude, inadequate knowledge, or lack of skill. On the other hand, if you bring high levels of energy, knowledge, and skill in addition to positive attitudes, your teaching is likely to be both effective and satisfying.

10

Assessment of the Teaching Situation

Once assessments of the teacher and learner have been made, the teaching situation must be assessed in terms of both resources and support.

RESOURCES

The resources involved in a patient teaching situation include people, time, space, money, and materials.

People

People are without doubt the most important resource. Effective teaching can take place in crowded quarters, with few if any teaching materials, despite noise and pressures of time IF the people involved are knowledgeable, skillful, concerned, and committed to patient teaching. Persons who are likely to prove helpful to the nurse are, first of all, consultants and specialists within the field of nursing. The clinical nurse specialist in cancer nursing, the nurse in charge of the pain clinic, the nurse with advanced preparation in the care of ostomy patients, or one of the nurses from the orthopedic unit may help you plan to meet the teaching needs of your patient.

It will be your responsibility to initiate the contact with a resource person. As you discover and work with a variety of specialists and consultants, you may find it helpful to keep a list of names and phone numbers to which you can refer as the need arises. This may be especially useful in relatively small communities in which there may be no published listing of agencies and resource people. It will be your responsibility to discover or develop working relationships that are effective and economical of everyone's time. In some instances the specialist may interact directly with your patient; most of the time, however, the consultant or specialist will work through you rather than personally teaching the patient. The task of a consultant is to help you to help your patient—it is not to take over the care of your patient.

If you need help that does not seem to be available, it is important to make your need known to persons in positions of authority, because many consultant or specialist positions are created in response to a demand or need for the services. It is difficult for an administrator to justify a position in the budget if there has been no apparent demand for the services of a person in that position.

Before you seek help, you will need to feel comfortable with the notion that you are not, and cannot be, all-knowing, or all things to all people. It is unrealistic to expect that you will be able to deal effectively with each and every situation you encounter, or to deal equally well with all aspects of a given situation. You may feel very comfortable as you meet the physical needs of an adolescent who tried to commit suicide, but feel inept and unqualified to meet the psychological needs of that patient and his parents. It takes confidence and courage to acknowledge that you do not feel qualified in a given area, and that you are actively seeking help, but it is only through the use of appropriate resources that you will be able to meet the teaching needs of your patients. In addition to nurses who serve as resource persons to you, many persons from other disciplines can give invaluable assistance—a dental hygienist, nutritionist, physical therapist, social worker, physician, and so on. There is no need to expect yourself to be knowledgeable and competent in every aspect of the patient's therapy and rehabilitation. Your task is to be knowledgeable and skilled in nursing, and then to help the patient to avail himself of the services of appropriate resource persons.

Time

Time is perhaps the second most important resource, for without it, you can do very little. It is probably true that in most agencies today, little or no time is set aside specifically for teaching. Few public health visits are made solely for the purpose of teaching, not because the staff is unwilling or not concerned, but because of problems related to payment for the nurse's time. So, in a large percentage of teaching situations, the nurse finds herself having to integrate patient teaching into other aspects of patient care. This may be very effective, but it does mean that you need to develop assessment and teaching skills that will enable you to establish a teaching situation QUICKLY, often while you are simultaneously attending to physical needs. You may not have time to sit down and write out objectives and detailed plans for teaching each patient, but once you have acquired the basic skills of teaching, you will be able to make your plans en route to the patient's home, to make notes about possible teaching needs as you listen to report or read the patient's chart. You can establish a climate in which five minutes at a patient's bedside can result in significant learning. Time certainly affects the quantity and quality of teaching, but lack of time is no excuse for failure to teach.

Space

Space and related aspects of the physical environment are important resources for learning. In many teaching situations a private space is critical. Depending upon the patient's diagnosis and prognosis, the patient's need for privacy may overshadow other considerations, such as adequate light and heat, minimal noise, and comfortable chairs. The patient who is learning to irrigate a colostomy, or the adolescent who is trying to learn to cope with an alcoholic parent, needs the privacy of a separate place shared for the moment with the nurse only.

In other situations the space provided is very much part of the message. If the Business and Professional Women's Club has been invited to your agency for a class, the space should be as light, airy, comfortable, and attractive as possible, because any space or environment that is markedly different from their everyday working space might prove distracting and detract from the class presentation. On the other hand, some people might find the space provided by the ultramodern chrome and plastic community room of a prestigious bank unsettling, lacking in warmth, and highly impersonal, regardless of the carefully prepared class or discussion. Whenever possible, the space you select should reflect the assessment you make of the needs of your learner. A small auditorium may provide the right degree of formality and importance for one group of learners, a corner of a laundromat may seem practical and convenient to another group, while her own bedroom may seem safest to a troubled teenager. If private space is limited, as in some acute care facilities, you may need to use an empty room on the unit, a conference room, or even the unit kitchen for patient teaching.

Money and Materials

The resources of money and materials are usually interrelated. Most agencies with large and extensive supplies of educational materials usually have a generous educational budget. There are exceptions, however. Many nurses are adept at obtaining free materials from drug companies, supply houses, commercial firms, and interested persons. It is possible to borrow film strips, video tapes, booklets, sample equipment, and many other types of educational materials. The local Cancer Society, for example, has many educational aids that can be borrowed for individual or group use. In some places, careful planning and purchasing by each of a group of agencies reduces duplication of materials and makes it easier to borrow materials back and forth.

SUPPORT

Of all the types and kinds of support relevant to patient teaching, five types will be discussed here. These are legal, administrative, medical, colleagueal, and familial support.

Legal Support

The nurse practice acts in some states include teaching in the legal definition of nursing. Therefore, in some situations teaching is not only supported—it is mandated by law. It is not an optional activity.

Administrative Support

While there may be few, if any, agencies or institutions that forbid patient teaching, many inhibit it by withholding support. Some institutions whose published philosophy of patient care makes reference to patient teaching may in fact fail to support and implement the concept of patient teaching. In assessing administrative support, you might ask, among other things, the following question: Does patient teaching have a high or low priority in this institution? This question may be answered by assessing the following areas.

Staffing. Is the staff adequate to permit each nurse time for teaching her patient? Are the work loads and assignments reasonable with respect to teaching? Is there continuity in assignments so that a nurse is able to teach a patient over a period of time?

Space. Must all teaching be done at the bedside, or are there a variety of spaces available in which the nurse may teach a single patient or a small group?

Rewards. What reward or reinforcement is given for effective patient teaching? Is any recognition given for creative or innovative teaching? On a very basic level, do head nurses and supervisors appear pleased when they observe a nurse sitting with a patient, teaching him, or do they, verbally or nonverbally, seem to disapprove?

Inservice education. Is assistance provided in the form of training programs, workshops on teaching techniques, conferences on new methods, and so on?

Materials. Are funds budgeted for the purchase or preparation of educational materials, such as booklets, pamphlets, posters?

Expectations. Are nurses expected to teach? Is it a regular, anticipated intervention important in its own right? Or must teaching be combined with some other activity in order to be acceptable?

Medical Support

What is the attitude of the physician in the situation? Is he an enthusiastic advocate of patient teaching by nurses? Is he neutral?— saying, in effect, "It's OK with me, teach if you want to, but it isn't really necessary." Or does he actively oppose the teaching of his patients by anyone other than himself? It is possible to teach effectively without support, such as when the physician is neutral, but not in the face of active opposition. While you may feel that you have an equally valid position, and that learning certain information or skills is essential to the patient's future well-being, you must consider carefully the possible consequences of any actions you may take. If you proceed to teach the patient, regardless of the physician's attitudes, the patient may be caught in the middle in an intenable position. It may seem that he is being forced to take sides, to choose between his physician and his nurse. You may feel that your actions are professionally correct, and yet they may seriously jeopardize the doctor-patient relationship and trust, which may be one of the essential aspects of the patient's therapy. It may be that all you should do is to support the patient in any attempts he may make to seek information from the doctor. You can teach the patient how to make the most of each interaction with the physician, such as writing down questions ahead of time, asking for clarification of things that are unclear, and being assertive enough to say, "Wait a minute, I need to talk to you." You can explain that he does have a right to know (42).

You do have a responsibility to further the cause of patient teaching, in behalf both of the nursing profession and of all patients, but this conflict should be resolved between nurses and physicians without involving a specific patient, whose situation may be worsened by the accompanying stress and tension. If the teaching needed is applicable to a group of patients, one strategy is to start a program for patients whose physicians approve. If the program is effective, those patients will promote it and others will ask permission to participate.

You may, upon occasion, be caring for a patient who is well aware of the discrepancy between the positions of his nurse and his physician, who is confident of his rights and strong enough to cope with any type of likely confrontation. You may, after careful consideration and discussion with the patient, decide to proceed with certain aspects of patient teaching, with full knowledge of the risk you are taking.

Colleagueal Support

Do your colleagues value patient teaching? If they do, they are likely to be interested in your methods and techniques, to encourage you when you encounter difficulties, and to follow through should one of them be assigned on your day off to a patient who has a rather urgent need to learn a specific skill or acquire certain information. If your colleagues do not value teaching as an integral part of nursing, the time and energy you invest in it may seem unnecessary or inappropriate to them.

Time spent in patient teaching may be viewed as time wasted or, in extreme situations, as shirking your "duties." You may seem to be violating group norms, if coffee breaks and informal conversation are the accepted use of time not spent in specifically ordered patient care. Your approach and your communication skills will determine whether your interest and enthusiasm for patient teaching acts as an incentive and example for your colleagues, or whether your behavior tends to alienate you from some of the staff.

Familial Support

Whenever possible, it is important that you assess the family support system before you attempt to plan for patient teaching. You need to assess the possible effect of the patient's condition on the rest of the family, and to determine the extent to which the patient is dependent upon another person or persons for some aspect of the behavior you hope to teach. It is both nonproductive and frustrating to spend time and energy helping a patient learn something that he can never fully use because of some constraint within his family system. For example, the pregnant teenager may become knowledgeable and motivated to seek adequate nutrition for herself and her unborn baby from state or federal food plans but be prevented from doing so by a father who, angered by her pregnancy, will not permit her to accept "welfare" to obtain the food supplements that he cannot or will not buy.

You will need to assess the relationship of the patient (the named or identified learner) to other persons who may in fact be the more critical learners. Such persons may include the family decision maker, the person in power or with authority, the one who manages the family budget, or the person who normally receives and processes similar information. One nurse had the experience of repeatedly trying to teach a patient how to adjust her diet. The woman kept saying, "The children will be home from school soon," "The children will be home from school soon." The nurse belatedly discovered that the oldest daughter, a high school student, was the person who in essence "managed" her mother's diabetic regimen. So the teaching had to be repeated with the daughter present, as she was the gatekeeper of that type of knowledge and information for that family.

If the family is experiencing a great deal of stress, for example in coping with the care of a parent on home dialysis, the anxiety of a school-age child and his subsequent behavior may prove disruptive to all normal interaction within the family. In such a situation, the child is one of the primary learners, and an essential task of the nurse is to teach the child to cope with his own feelings about his parent's illness and pending death. Family support may involve a willingness to allow an adolescent to learn how to manage essential aspects of his own condition, or a willingness to relinquish space, such as temporarily giving up the dining room for a first-floor bedroom for grandmother as she recuperates after a fractured hip. Support may be a commitment to an altered budget that will permit therapy for a member of the family, especially if there is a choice, if the condition is not actually life-threatening. It may be a willingness to give of time and energy in order to assume responsibility for additional or different tasks related to the patient's condition.

Ideally, the nurse should meet the various members of the family and assess the varying degrees of support. When this is not possible, a beginning assessment can be made by asking a variety of questions, such as: "How do you expect your _____ (husband, wife, child) will react to _____ (your diet, your need to be on the first floor, or whatever)?" "What kind of changes will this _____ make in your day-to-day routines?" "Who is most likely to help you with _____?" Of all the initial data to be collected, information related to the patient's family system is among the most important. Without a basic knowledge of the patient's support systems, you may base your approach on incorrect assumptions, which can lead to faulty and ineffective teaching.

SUMMARY

The initial phase of any teaching is an assessment of the learner, the teacher, and the teaching-learning situation. This assessment may range from a quick appraisal before a spontaneous teaching interaction to a full-scale research project to assess the needs, attitudes, location, numbers, and so on of clients for a community education project. Regardless of the scope or nature of the anticipated patient teaching or health education, the assessment phase is the keystone for subsequent success or failure.

THE TEACHING-LEARNING PROCESS

PLANNING

11

Objectives

THE NEED FOR AND USES OF OBJECTIVES

If a person has unlimited time, money, and other necessary resources, he can afford to drift in search of a career, education, companion, or perfect vacation. If, however, one of his resources becomes limited, he must narrow his search in order to complete it before that resource runs out. For example, a person with unlimited resources who wants to buy a vacation home may inspect homes in Hawaii, Monte Carlo, the Rocky Mountains, Florida, and Alaska, spending a few weeks in each location. If, however, his time or money becomes limited, he may decide to have a real estate agent submit photographs of three choice homes in each location, and he can then choose one or two to actually visit. Another way he can limit the search is to state the activities he hopes to pursue during a vacation. A preference for lying in the sun will focus attention on Florida or Hawaii, and if lying in the sun is coupled with a desire to learn surfing, the search is further narrowed to Hawaii. Rather than consider every available vacation home in Hawaii, the searcher needs to establish criteria for an acceptable home, including price range, size, proximity to major cities, accessibility (by bus, car, plane, or helicopter), and so on. Once a realtor knows the standards of acceptability, he can proceed to locate vacation homes within the desired range.

So it is with many activities of our everyday lives. If we have lots of time, energy, money, and other resources, we can engage in random, ill-defined, almost purposeless activities. If, however, we are interested in conserving one or more of our resources, we need to limit our activities and to establish criteria for their selection. In patient teaching and health education, resources usually are limited. In an acute care setting, time and energy are often in short supply. In an extended care or community health setting, you may have more time in the sense that you have a more prolonged contact with the patient and family, but money and energy are limited. Community health nurses often find that teaching is feasible only in situations in which treatment or physical care is needed, because some insurance programs and other sources of funding will not pay for visits in which the sole intervention is teaching. In health education programs for the public, many resources are limited. In public school programs, a major restriction is time. You may be allotted a specific number classes over a specified period of weeks, with no leeway whatsoever. When you present material through the mass media, your message in a newspaper or magazine is limited in space, and your message on radio or television is limited in time. Therefore, since the resources for patient teaching are usually limited, and since there is often no second chance, it behooves each nurse to make the most of each opportunity and to decide what can best be accomplished with the resources available.

The process of describing what can realistically be accomplished in a given teaching situation follows a careful assessment of the learner, the teacher, and the situation. The description of what is to be accomplished has been given a variety of names, including purposes, goals, and objectives. Purposes are often stated in broad, general terms. Goals are less general, while objectives are narrow and specific. Purposes and goals often represent long-range intentions and aspirations, but objectives usually represent immediate or short-range outcomes, outcomes that are related to a specific learning experience.

Well-stated objectives are difficult to write, but their usefulness far outweighs the stress of learning to write them. Only the basic concepts of writing objectives will be presented in this book. For more information, see the bibliography.

EDUCATIONAL OBJECTIVES

According to Robert Mager, each educational objective has three parts: the behavior, criteria, and conditions. If all three parts are present, an objective may be used as a basis for planning, for teaching, and for evaluation.

An objective attempts to answer three questions:

1. What should the learner be able to do? (the behavior)
2. How well should he be able to do it? (the criteria)
3. Under what conditions should he be able to do it? (the condition)

The Behavior

To be useful, an educational objective must describe a behavior that can be observed and measured. Such an objective is called, appropriately enough, a behavioral objective. The objective must contain an active verb, which indicates what the learner will do if he successfully meets the objective. He may run a mile, point to three objects, assemble a model, draw a diagram, recite a poem, or perform any of hundreds of other actions. These actions are all observable, in contrast to activities such as to think, ponder, understand, contemplate, or know. *An observable behavior is one that can be seen or heard by another person.* Nonobservable behaviors may indicate that learning has taken place, but such learning cannot be readily evaluated. Only the learner can tell if it has taken place. Much of the learning that results from the patient's contact with you will be of this nature, and in the long run, this nonobservable learning may be the most significant to the patient. For several reasons, however, you need to be able to measure the learning that has taken place.

First, behavioral objectives facilitate feedback about your teaching. If learning has taken place, that knowledge will give reward and satisfaction, which you need. If learning is not taking place, you will know that you need to reassess the situation and modify your approach or expectations.

In many situations, evaluation is important because the effectiveness of patient teaching or a health education program determines the extent of resources that will be made available for future programs. It stands to reason that a successful teaching program or project is more likely to be supported and funded in the future than one that resulted in no measurable learning. Which brings us full circle to behavioral objectives. If you do not have objectives for your teaching, you cannot tell if the patient has achieved the desired or expected learning. The learning cannot be evaluated, because neither he nor you have stated what was desired or expected. The motorist who embarks upon a business trip may pass through many interesting, scenic places, but if he does not know the name of his destination, he cannot tell when he has arrived. The patient may learn a wide variety of interesting and useful facts and skills and yet miss the most significant learning simply because neither you nor he knew what it was.

The behavioral portion of an educational objective is a statement of the learner's ability to do something at the conclusion of the learning experience. Some of these abilities are very narrow and specific, such as the ability to walk with crutches. Others are much broader, such as the ability to maintain a prescribed diet while eating in college dining rooms and restaurants.

The Conditions

Most learning results in the ability to perform a task under one rather specific set of circumstances, but not under others. For example, a child might learn how to ride a bicycle safely on the streets of his suburban neighborhood, but he would not be expected to be able to do so on a major highway or through the business district of a large city. An objective for a freshman nursing student might include the behavior "to feed a patient." If no conditions were stated, one might assume that she was expected to be able to feed any patient. This is unrealistic. She might be able to feed a convalescent patient, but until she received further teaching, she could not be expected to feed an infant who had just had surgery for a cleft palate, a patient who was nauseated from chemotherapy, or a patient whose swallowing reflex had been impaired.

A young girl may be able to bathe her baby with the support of the nurse in the hospital but may be unable to manage the same task under the critical eye of her mother or mother-in-law. If you discover, in your assessment of the learning situation, that the girl may have difficulty at home, you may need to help her learn to bathe the baby in the home setting, and to help the girl learn to cope with the mother. One thing is certain: the fact that the girl can bathe the baby comfortably in the hospital does not guarantee her ability to do so at home.

Your task is to determine the conditions under which the patient or family will actually be doing the desired activity, and then teach for performance under those conditions. The objectives for the learning should reflect that situation. For example, if the patient will be caring for his colostomy in the shared bathroom of his rooming house, that situation needs to be simulated as closely as possible when you are teaching. He is ill prepared for discharge if he knows how to care for himself only in the privacy of a well-equipped hospital bathroom.

Often the conditions are stated as "givens." The objective may read "Given (the conditions), the learner will (the behavior). For example: Given a sterile dressing tray, the student will _____, Given regular supervision by a private pediatrician, the mother will _____. Given the assistance of a home health aide, the patient's wife will be able to _____.

Ideally, objectives are written out. This helps to insure *clarity* (so that each objective is thought through, clearly and logically), *consistency* (so that you can remember and carry out the plans you have made with each patient), and *continuity* (so that other members of the staff can contribute to the patient's learning when you are not present. In your day-to-day nursing practice, often it may not be possible to sit down and write out your objectives, but you can think each one through carefully. Ask yourself, "What should this patient be able to do?" and then "Under what conditions, or under what circumstances, should he be able to do it?" These two questions will help you formulate the behavior and conditions of each objective.

The Criteria

Most of us can well remember the taunting cry of childhood, "Yeah? Who says?" In many ways this cry is analogous to the criteria of an objective, for each asks, "By what standards?" "By whose authority?" and "To whose satisfaction?" The criteria indicate how well the task must be performed to be considered acceptable. In a math exam, what degree of accuracy is expected? 100%? or 65%? In giving range-of-motion exercises, what constitutes full range of motion? The textbook description? The patient's comfort? The physiotherapist's recommendation?

The phrase, "according to Hoyle," represents an example of criteria or standards. Just as Hoyle can be designated the authority for rules of card games, so can other authorities or criteria be designated as the standard of desired performance for any behavior. Some behaviors must be 100% perfect: there can be, for example, no deviation or error in sterile technique. At the other extreme, the criteria may rest within the learner. The criteria may be the learner's comfort or satisfaction, as determined by the learner. The person who fears heights or water or spiders may have set an objective to work with a therapist until he feels comfortable in the formerly threatening situation. Of course it would be possible to monitor his physiological responses to the threat, and to use changes in pulse rate, respiration, and galvanic skin response as indicators of progress toward the goal, but in this instance it is simpler, more natural, and probably more accurate to use the patient's perception of comfort as a criterion of effective learning.

The majority of objectives have criteria that lie between the perfect performance that is necessary for sterile technique and the inner criteria of comfort. Many objectives state an authority or standard against which the learner's performance can be measured. The criteria portion of an objective often includes a phrase such as: "as listed in the hospital diet sheet," "as described in the agency manual," or "as demonstrated by the physiotherapist." Sometimes the criteria specify that an acceptable performance must be completed in a certain length of time or a specified number of attempts.

Ideally, criteria should be written and shared with the learner before the learning experience. Then he not only knows what behavior is expected of him, but he also knows its quality. He knows the basis upon which he will be judged and has a standard whereby he can evaluate his own performance. Even if the criteria are not available in written form, they can be communicated orally to the patient with similar results. The learner knows what is expected of him, and misunderstandings or disagreements related to achievement are minimized. If criteria are not shared and are not made explicit, some version of the following dialogue is likely to ensue: "But I did it!" "Yes, but you didn't do it right." "Well, you never said I couldn't do it that way." "That's because I assumed that anybody would do it this way. It's the way everyone here does it."

Let us summarize the points made so far. There are three parts to an objective: the behavior (what will the learner be able to do?), the conditions (under what circumstances will he be able to do?), and the criteria (how well will he be able to do it?). When you can, it is useful to write out your objectives, because the process of writing requires a careful thinking through of all three parts until the behavior, conditions, and criteria are clearly and concisely spelled out. In many instances it is neither possible nor appropriate to write out each objective, and it becomes doubly important for the you to develop the skill of formulating objectives mentally.

Objectives are important because they permit feedback about learning. If the learner has met the objectives, effective learning has taken place, and this knowledge serves as a necessary reward and reinforcement for teacher and learner. If the objectives were not met, learning may be inadequate, and this feedback suggests that the teacher reassess her approach and/or her expectations for the learner. (See Chapter 16 for discussion of feedback, reward, and reinforcement.)

MUTUAL DEVELOPMENT OF OBJECTIVES

Time is one of your most important resources, and since it is often in short supply, it behooves you to use it wisely. One way to do so is make sure that the objectives for patient teaching are mutually acceptable to both you and the patient. If the patient participates in developing the objectives, there will be less question of their acceptability. This premise must be validated, however, because a nurse represents AUTHORITY to many patients, and they will follow your lead in developing objectives as readily as they will follow directions about a treatment.

A patient may try to be a "good patient" by complying with a routine or procedure in the hospital that he has neither the intention nor the ability to follow at home. The patient who agreeably participates in a discussion of low-salt diets may be thinking to himself, "Lady, you're wasting your time. I live with my sister and she'll fix the meals just the way she has for the past 25 years." The teaching, in this situation, is a waste of your time and his unless it follows mutually acceptable and mutually significant objectives.

In a conjunctive approach to learning, the teacher and learner assume joint responsibility for the learner's education. The learner is an active participant in the educational process. He makes his needs known, gives feedback to the teacher, and participates in the evaluation of his progress and performance. The same approach is valid for patient teaching. The patient is likely to learn more effectively if he has an opportunity to participate in the planning, implementation, and evaluation of his learning. This participation includes the development of objectives.

It would probably be most unwise for you to permit the patient to assume *full* control of his learning for a variety of reasons. He lacks the knowledge to identify the aspects of his condition that may be critical or even life-threatening, his psychological status at the moment may interfere with logical thought and planning, or he may lack the energy and motivation to seek learning experiences. In other words, he may be too ill, depressed, upset, tired, or discouraged to try to figure out what he needs to learn in order to improve his lot. Therefore, it is not fair to dismiss your responsibility in the name of a conjunctive approach to learning by saying, "If he had wanted to know, he would have asked," or words to that effect.

In a conjunctive approach, you have a professional responsibility to initiate the teaching-learning process. You do so by developing an atmosphere conducive to learning and by making the initial assessments of yourself, the patient, and the situation.

Once the assessments have been made, you enter the phase of goal setting, a time when purposes and objectives are established. This phase of the teaching-learning process corresponds to the diagnostic phase of nursing process. At present, there is no terminology or classification system for this phase of teaching; there is simply an emphasis upon clear, accurate, and concise objectives. In the future you may be able to formulate a precise Learning Diagnosis or develop a Statement of Learning Needs. The nature of the objectives depends upon input from the patient, physician, family, nurse, and any other persons who are significant within the health care and family systems. Your input consists of a knowledge of what the patient *needs*, and the patient's input consists of what he *wants*. Sometimes there is considerable overlap of input from patient and nurse; at other times the distance between them is great. Your skill as a teacher will be reflected in your ability to integrate your input and the patient's into a meaningful set of objectives.

You will eventually develop your own approach to this process, but initially you might try the following one. As you conclude the assessment phase, you might say something such as: "From what you have told me, it seems that you are concerned about your _____ and _____. And as I see it, you are interested in _____ and _____. Is this right?" ". . . . ."

"Based on this, you seem to want to learn _____ and _____. From my experience, I can pretty well predict that you will need to know how to _____ and _____. Given these needs and interests, let's decide where to start. Which ones seem most important to you?" ". . . . ."

As you and the patient work to develop a meaningful set of objectives, you may find it helpful to couple the desired behavior with the patient's reason for wanting to learn it. The format "*to learn* . . . . . . *in order to* . . . ." is often useful. For example, "I want to learn to use a walker so that I can get to the bathroom at home when everyone is at work." If you know the patient's reason for wanting to learn something, you are able to put that task into a context that may indicate a need for more teaching. The patient who needs a walker to get to the bathroom may need to learn how to manipulate himself and the walker if the bathroom is extremely small or the toilet is relatively inaccessible.

OBJECTIVES AND CONTINUITY OF TEACHING

Because of the fragmentation created by our current health care delivery system it is imperative that the patient be involved as much as possible in setting goals and objectives for his own learning. Since he may be transferred from unit to unit, and from facility to facility, he may be the only person who is aware of his objectives and progress to date. A patient may move from an intensive care unit to a progressive care unit, then to a regular medical-surgical unit within an acute care setting, then to an extended care facility and finally home. Despite these moves, the patient and his family may be able to structure for themselves some kind of continuity IF they were involved from the beginning with the setting of objectives. This responsibility for continuity should not be delegated or deliberately shifted onto the patient, however. It is a nursing responsibility, and some nurses are actively seeking innovative ways to insure continuity of teaching as the patient moves from unit to unit and from facility to facility. In situations in which nursing has not yet assumed this responsibility, or has not yet implemented an effective plan for doing so, the use of well-stated objectives can help your patient gain at least minimal control over his own learning.

Some patients in an acute care setting do not move from unit to unit. Even so, your opportunities for any long-range teaching may be severely limited by the shortness of many hospitalizations. In order to facilitate any extended teaching, such as teaching a newly diagnosed patient with hypertension, or the parents of a premature infant, you will need to contact the community health nurse or clinic nurse who may follow the patient. A request for follow-up teaching may be part of the agency's referral system, but referrals usually have more to do with physical care and physician's orders than with patient teaching. It is important that a referral include the behavioral objectives relevant to the patient's needs and an assessment of his learning to date.

To summarize briefly, behavioral objectives provide direction for both teaching the patient and evaluating his learning. These objectives, which should be mutually acceptable to both you and the patient, facilitate continuity of teaching despite changes in staff or environment.

12

The Domains of Learning

The behaviors and actions of man were divided by early Greek philosophers into three groups, and this same threefold division is still evident today. We speak of knowledge, attitudes, and skills, or of thinking, feeling, and acting. With reference to educational objectives, we speak of the cognitive, affective, and psychomotor domains or classifications. These domains are significant because the characteristics of learning within each domain influence the selection of teaching methods and the method of evaluation.

An objective in the *cognitive* domain deals with the recall or recognition of information and the development of intellectual abilities and skills. Objectives in the *affective* domain describe changes in feeling, tone, emotion, interest, and attitude and are related to values as well as degrees of acceptance or rejection. The psychomotor domain emphasizes muscular or motor skills, tasks that require coordination and dexterity and often some manipulation of materials or objects.

The nature of each domain is indicated by the verbs commonly associated with it. For example:

Cognitive: remembering, recalling, interpreting, analyzing, problem solving, calculating, deciding, thinking.

Affective: feeling, valuing, accepting, desiring, seeking.

Psychomotor: walking, lifting, holding, turning, balancing.

Within each of these three domains is a hierarchy of educational objectives. For the purposes of this book, however, I will refer to each domain as a whole.

WRITING OBJECTIVES IN EACH DOMAIN

Objectives in the *psychomotor domain* are the easiest to write in behavioral terms because the action is obvious. The verbs are specific and the behavior is easily observed. Examples of psychomotor objectives are: to give an injection, walk with crutches, apply hot packs, read a thermometer, or bathe a baby.

If you encounter difficulty in teaching or evaluating a psychomotor skill, it may be that the skill you are trying to teach is composed of several component skills, each of which should be taught and evaluated separately. For example, the objective "to breast feed a baby" is composed of at least three subobjectives, each of which needs to be taught (unless it has already been reached). These objectives would include being able to prepare and keep the nipples in good condition, to handle the baby, and to actually nurse the baby. Each skill is essential. If the mother has never picked up or held an infant, she is likely to need help in doing so before she will be able to position the baby for feeding.

Sometimes it is helpful to state a subobjective as follows: "To learn . . . in preparation for. . . ." This format indicates clearly that the objective is a contributing objective and makes explicit its relationship to a main objective.

Objectives in the *cognitive domain* are harder to write because you cannot observe the actual behavior, you can only infer its occurrence from the product that results. You cannot watch a person think or remember or calculate, but you can observe him make a list, take a test, describe an event, or present a case. You will need to avoid all abstract terms such as to know, to realize, and to understand, and substitute a verb that will give an action or product that you can see or hear. There must be a behavior that can be observed if the objective is to be considered behavioral.

Examples of cognitive objectives would include: State the name and dose of current medications, describe the characteristics of a two-year-old child, list the seven warning signs of cancer, and describe the safety measures needed for an elderly person who is returning home after fracturing his hip.

Objectives in the *affective domain* are the hardest to write in behavioral terms. It is difficult to avoid using phrases such as to value, to appreciate, and to believe, and substitute words that indicate a measurable behavior. Robert Mager uses *approach behaviors*—actions that indicate the learner is coming toward the desired behavior—as evidence that the learner is beginning to value it positively, that he sees some worth in it. Examples of behavioral objectives in the affective domain might include: verbalizes fears about surgery to parents or nurse, adheres to prescribed diet, seeks support from members of group, keeps clinic appointments, and complies with medical regimen.

Since attitudes and feelings are often difficult to change, the learner may seem slow to reach objectives in the affective domain. His progress will be easier to support and evaluate if the behavior in each objective is small enough to accomplish and measure in a relatively short time. An objective that requires a patient to "adopt and sustain a life style compatible with the treatment of hypertension" cannot be attained for many months or even years. A more useful objective would be "to do one thing each day for the next month to minimize the effects of an identified stressor." Both you and the patient can note progress toward the second objective, and you can modify your teaching as needed in order to help the patient accomplish it.

TEACHING IN EACH DOMAIN

Psychomotor Domain

Teaching in the psychomotor domain usually requires a demonstration plus considerable feedback and opportunities for practice. Elements of the other two domains are usually present in varying degrees, especially in the early phase of learning a psychomotor skill. Initially, the learner needs an explanation—a theoretical or cognitive basis for the motor skill he is to learn. If he is fearful, apprehensive, resentful, or resistant, extensive teaching in the affective domain may be needed before any attempt is made to proceed with the psychomotor objective.

Some of the assessments that must be made have been mentioned in the chapters on assessment of the learner and readiness to learn. Specific assessments would include an evaluation of strength, dexterity, coordination, and sense of balance. Optimal eyesight must be insured through good lighting and eyeglasses (freshly cleaned) as needed.

If equipment is to be used, it should be adjusted whenever possible to the height and size of the patient.

One assessment that is quite specific to the psychomotor domain is that of clothing. In general, the patient should wear comfortable supportive shoes instead of slippers. Street clothes are preferable to gowns and robes for three reasons: 1) the patient avoids becoming tangled up in folds of robe or gown (as when trying to learn to transfer from wheelchair to toilet), 2) the patient can learn a skill more easily if there are no loose sleeves to contaminate a sterile field or get caught in a mechanical device, and 3) you can evaluate the patient's performance more readily if his movements are not obscured by a robe (as during crutch walking). If street clothes are not feasible, pajamas are preferable to a long gown, and a tailored robe is preferable to a fluffy, flowing one for a woman.

Two final assessments are needed with respect to the psychomotor domain: "How does he feel about learning this skill?" and "How does he learn best?"

The way a person feels about learning a motor skill is influenced by his perception of himself as being clumsy or adept. The person who views himself as clumsy must worry about your reaction to his lack of coordination in addition to being concerned about learning the motor skill. Fear of operating mechanical or electrical equipment may range from mild apprehension in some persons to near panic in others, especially if the equipment is attached to a person and there is even the remotest possibility of his being injured. Some persons are very fearful of any procedure involving oxygen. No matter what you think of such reactions, it is important that you accept the person's feelings about learning the motor skill as both valid and significant, and that you provide the support needed as the person tries to learn the task.

The patient's perception of how he learns best is important in teaching a psychomotor skill. He will probably be able to identify himself as a *tell-me* or a *show-me* person. A tell-me person is verbally oriented and often prefers to read a set of instructions for himself and then proceed to follow them. The most pronounced tell-me person I have encountered was the daughter of a friend who was not profiting from swimming lessons. Her comment was, "If they'd only tell me what I'm supposed to be doing!" Her father tried to explain that you don't *tell* a person how to swim, but she insisted. So, her father explained what each arm and leg motion was supposed to accomplish, what was to happen each time she lifted her head, and so on. After being *told*, she promptly learned to swim.

Others are equally intense show-me persons. My mother crochets well but simply cannot interpret the directions. I do not crochet well, but if I read the directions and show her, mother is able to complete the pattern without difficulty.

Ask your patient how he learns best and how he would like to proceed. His self-knowledge and insights are likely to be most helpful as you prepare to teach a psychomotor skill.

Cognitive Domain

Teaching in the cognitive domain usually involves the transmission of information from one person to another person or to a group. Information usually is presented directly through an explanation or lecture, although a variety of media may be used.

The assessments that are specific to the cognitive domain would include those of general intellectual abilities, such as verbal skills and literacy. Specific assessments would include the abilities needed to reach each objective. For example, an objective that requires an elderly patient to "state the name, dose, and main effects of each drug you are currently taking" might seem reasonable to you, but overwhelming to the patient if he has not tried to memorize anything in years, and especially if he has recently been plagued by a failing memory. He may truly be unable to memorize and recite the information. Rather than subject him to the frustration of trying, and the humiliation of failing, you may need to teach him to post the information in several places at home, and carry it with him at all times.

If your patient seems unable to meet the cognitive objectives, reassess his ability. Confusion, or decrease in mental clarity or level of alertness, may be caused by a reaction to drugs or a change in the patient's physical condition. Whatever the cause, the difficulty must be corrected before you can proceed. If it cannot be corrected, you will need to modify the cognitive objectives.

Affective Domain

Teaching in the affective domain usually seeks to change or at least modify an attitude or emotional response, to create interest, or to nurture a tendency to act in a certain way. This change is most likely to result from interaction within a small supportive group, or as a result of an extensive one-to-one interaction with a person who holds the desired attitude or emotional response. Affective learning does not result from a lecture or explanation.

Teaching in the affective domain may need to precede teaching in the other two domains, especially in situations in which the learner has strong feelings about the subject or skill to be learned. A person who is in the throes of a strong emotion is unable to attend to anything else until his emotional response has been dealt with.

A change in attitude takes place slowly; it cannot be forced. It is usually futile to try to deal directly with an attitude, to confront the person and ask or demand that he change his attitude.

The reason for wanting to change an attitude is to change a given behavior that it influences. You are likely to be more successful in changing the attitude if you structure situations that will elicit those behaviors that would be evident if the person had the desired attitude. It is easier to change a behavior than an attitude, and it is appropriate and effective to do so because the changed behavior will be followed by a changed attitude. Putting this another way, it is easier for a person to act his way into a new way of thinking than it is for him to think his way into a different way of behaving. For example, if a person with a terminally ill relative feels warmth and emotional support from a group of people, he is likely to return and seek out the group. This will happen even though he had previously characterized himself as a loner and had rejected the idea of emotional support when you talked with him about the need for it through the months to come. This change in behavior will be followed by a change in attitude. The behavior of accepting and then seeking support from a group will be followed by a new attitude toward the value and worth of group interaction.

13

Selection of Content and Method

Content is elusive because it is an abstract concept and, strictly speaking, you cannot *select* content at all. If anyone were to ask you to select the content for teaching a newly diagnosed diabetic, your answer should be: "That's impossible—there is no such thing as the content for a newly diagnosed diabetic!" Content is derived from objectives, and objectives are specific to each patient. The needs, and therefore the objectives, are very different for a seven-year-old girl whose care will be managed by her parents, a 16-year-old athlete whose only concern at the moment is the effect that diabetes and "needles" will have upon his Olympic aspirations, and a 35-year-old man who is preoccupied with thoughts of complications such as amputation and blindness.

There may be some commonalities among the objectives for these three patients, just as the content for any number of newly diagnosed patients may have elements in common. That does not mean, however, that you could ever select the content for a newly diagnosed diabetic. Nevertheless, the term *selection of content* is in common use, and so it will be used in this book as a kind of imprecise shorthand.

INPUT FOR OBJECTIVES AND CONTENT

In patient teaching, the content to be learned consists of the knowledge, attitudes, and skills needed by the patient in order to attain the objectives he and the nurse have established. Input for the objectives and the resultant content comes from both professional and personal sources. Professional input comes from the nurse, physician, and other members of the health team. Personal input comes from the patient and his family.

Professional Input

Your knowledge and expertise, coupled with that of other members of the health team, provide the basis for patient teaching. Without this solid base of sound, accurate, factual knowledge, the content of your teaching would be flimsy indeed.

Input from nurse. Your contribution will be based in part upon your own experiences with other patients who have had similar conditions or problems, and in part upon the experiences of other nurses, which are available to you through professional journals and textbooks. These data enable you to hypothesize and to predict with a fair degree of accuracy some of the teaching that is likely to be needed by a given patient.

Input from physician. This information will be based upon the patient's diagnosis, prognosis, and treatment plan, the doctor's past experience with other patients, and what he has learned from his colleagues. It is important that both you and the physician draw freely upon your own experiences and the experiences of others, because such cumulative wisdom facilitates a rational, professional approach to teaching rather than a trial-and-error, start-from-scratch approach with each new patient.

Input from other members of the health team. In many instances neither you nor the physician will have all of the competencies needed to teach a particular patient. In such cases, the selection of content for that patient's teaching will be greatly influenced by the contributions of the physical therapist, nutritionist, rehabilitation specialist, psychiatric consultant, or any other member of the health care team.

Categories of Professional Input

The first step in selecting content for patient teaching is to separate those things that are necessary in order to meet the objectives from those things that are nice to know. Professional input can, and should, be divided into two categories: the content that is necessary for the protection, safety, and well-being of the patient, and the content that might be desirable, informative, and possibly useful. These distinctions are often difficult to make, because they change from time to time with a given patient, and from patient to patient. At the onset of an acute illness, the teaching needed may seem very limited in scope and depth, but any more information is superfluous and unnecessary for the patient's immediate needs. Later on, the information that was unnecessary at the onset of the illness becomes very necessary.

For example, the family of a patient admitted to the hospital with a massive stroke do not need to be taught about rehabilitation until it is known that the patient will recover and they are able to look to the future. As the patient and family begin to move toward objectives related to physical therapy, speech therapy, and other aspects of rehabilitation, you will need to select more content, which again is divided into what is necessary and what is nice to know. The patient and family need to know how to help prevent contractures; they do not need to know the terms *flexion* and *extension* in order to do this (the words *bend* and *straighten* will do). Some persons will want to know the correct terminology, and they certainly have the right to know, but it is not NECESSARY in terms of their being able to exercise the affected extremities.

Since your time with the patient and family is a precious commodity, it must be wisely used. It is important, therefore, to identify the minimum content that will enable the patient to reach the objectives that have been set. Once that content has been thoroughly learned, add MORE content if feasible. The selection of additional content will be influenced by the patient's readiness for more, and by your own available time and energy. In short, minimal teaching, effectively done, is better than presenting extensive material, little of which is learned or even necessary.

Responsibility for professional input.   The phrases *acts of commission* and *acts of omission* might well be applied to the selection of minimal content. It is easy to see how a nurse could be held liable if inaccurate information caused a patient to jeopardize his well-being, or if incorrect information caused him to do something that had a detrimental effect on his condition. On the other hand, it is equally reasonable that the nurse and physician be held accountable if they fail to give adequate information. For example, failure to teach a person who is on anticoagulant therapy that he should carry essential information in his wallet could result in grave consequences, if he were injured and taken, unconscious, to a nearby hospital for emergency surgery.

In some instances, the responsibility for failure to teach essential content must be shared by both doctor and nurse. In other situations, the responsibility must be born by the nurse alone, depending upon the nature of the content that was not taught.

Personal Input

Input from the patient will be based upon his desire to know and his fears or concerns, and will indicate what he wants to accomplish and how he expects to cope with his situation or condition. Input from the family will be based upon their response to the patient's situation or condition and will reveal, either directly or indirectly, some clues about the effect on the family. As members of the family indicate the things they want to know, or that they feel the patient should know, you will be able to assess the impact of the current situation on them and will discover ways in which you can teach them to cope more effectively.

The information sought by the patient may be almost exactly what he needs to know. He may ask, "What are the precautions I must take?" "What are the possible complications?" or "Are there any side effects to this drug?" In other situations, however, there may seem to be little relationship between the information the patient seeks and that which professional persons have indicated is necessary. In any event, both categories of information are important and must be included. The information the patient *must* know in order to meet the objectives that have been established, together with the information the patient *wants* to know, prescribes the content for patient teaching.

SELECTION OF METHOD

Given the assessments you have made, the objectives that have been developed, and the content that has been identified, the next step is to decide upon the method of teaching. The most commonly used methods are described in detail in the next chapter. Let us look now at the factors that will influence your choice of method.

Choosing a Method of Teaching

Your choice of a method for teaching your patient and his family depends on the factors described below.

Objectives.   The method of teaching is influenced not so much by the topic as by the objectives that have been set. For example, you might be asked to speak on sex education to two different groups. A straightforward, intellectual presentation of concepts related to sex education may be appropriate in meeting the objectives of the first group. With the second group, however, you may need to focus on helping two bitterly divided factions agree on a mutually acceptable approach to sex education in the elementary school. The topic and much of the content may be the same, but your method of teaching must be different.

Domains of learning. The selection of a method of teaching is influenced by the nature of the learning that is to take place, whether it is to be largely cognitive, affective, or psychomotor. Different methods are needed to impart information, change an attitude, and develop a skill.

The learners. Your choice of method will be influenced by the number of learners as well as by their age and capability. As an extreme example, the method of choice for teaching 30 intelligent persons will be significantly influenced if you know whether these 30 persons are third-graders or senior citizens.

Physical resources. Physical resources include money for publicity; brochures and other printed materials; audiovisual materials; and the comfort and privacy of the available space.

Time. Your selection of a method of teaching will be significantly affected by the constraints of time. You may prefer to teach each patient in an acute care setting individually and yet feel obliged to teach groups of patients to avoid repetition and save time.

The teacher. Last but definitely not least, the selection of a method of teaching depends on your own energy, capabilities, and preference. There is no *right* method in any given situation, and the best method is likely to be the one with which you feel most comfortable at that particular point in your career.

THE
TEACHING-LEARNING
PROCESS

IMPLEMENTATION

14

Methods of Teaching

In an ideal situation, your choice of teaching methods should be determined by your objectives and the nature of your material, as well as by the number and characteristics of the learners. In real life, your choice of method will also be influenced by the amount of space, time, and other resources available to you.

I will describe seven teaching methods that I think you will find useful in health education and patient teaching. There are numerous other methods, but these are the ones that you can use in your nursing practice and community activities without having to seek extensive funding, equipment, or administrative action.

LECTURE

The lecture is an effective method of group instruction. It is essentially a one-way communication from teacher to learners, with little or no input back to the teacher. It is highly efficient for two reasons. First, the material can be carefully organized and precisely timed so that each available minute is used to full advantage. In a group discussion, by contrast, the group may digress from the topic or waste time in diffuse or unfocused discussion. Second, with the use of closed-circuit television, microphones, and other audiovisual equipment, there is virtually no limit to the number of persons who can be reached by a single lecture. They can be seated in a huge hall or arena or in a number of separate rooms. It is even possible to lecture to a group of persons in a distant city via telephone, and the audience can participate in a question-and-answer period via telephone after the lecture. A lecture to a large group often eliminates repeating the same material to a number of small groups, with little or no decrease in learning.

Given that active involvement and participation increase learning, the lecturer must search for ways to promote active interaction between learner and content. This interaction occurs when the material is stimulating, thought provoking, and relevant, when it elicits an intellectual response from the learner. The content may be weighty and serious, but the presentation need never be dull or ponderous. When lecturing, you will need to seek a lively, personable, and interesting approach, which reflects your own ideas and perspective.

The lecture should represent a synthesis of ideas from a variety of sources rather than a recital of material from a single source, which learners could read for themselves. The material may be new, such as a report of the latest research on a topic, or you may present familiar material from a different perspective, possibly based upon your personal experiences or a case study.

If possible, give your first few lectures on topics that are very familiar to you so that your energy can be spent on achieving a comfortable and satisfying presentation rather than on acquiring new material, which may still be unfamiliar at the time of the lecture.

Preparation of the Lecture

The first step in preparation of a lecture is an assessment of the learners. Much of your data will come from the committee or person who asked you to speak to the group. If the information listed below is not volunteered, you will need to ask for it. You need to know the following:

1. The objectives.
   Why were you asked to speak, and what are you expected to accomplish?
2. The placement of your lecture in the series or schedule of programs.
   It makes a difference whether you are the first, middle, or last speaker of the series or course.
3. The content of any previous lectures.
   Is there any relationship between preceding lectures and your own? Are you expected to continue or develop a theme?
4. The number and characteristics of the learners.
   How many are expected? How were they recruited? Interest in the lecture may be different if attendance is voluntary rather than required, such as with a high school assembly. What are the general characteristics and background of the audience? You will prepare a lecture on hypertension quite differently for college students, retired businessmen, church women, and professional athletes.

Given answers to these and other questions you may choose to ask, you will be able to begin an overall assessment of the teaching situation.

Sometimes you can discover even more about the interests, knowledge, and motivation of your learners by taking a poll or survey of the group in advance of the lecture. If there is time, and if money is available from the group or agency that asked you to speak, you can develop and distribute a printed or dittoed questionnaire to help you determine the needs and interests of the potential audience, so that you can develop a lecture to meet their needs.

If you feel confident about your knowledge of the lecture material, and feel that you could modify it on the spot, you can obtain valuable clues about the audience's background and interest through a show of hands at the beginning of the lecture. You can ask questions ranging from "How many of you have heard the term . . .?" to "How many of you have ever known someone who has . . .?" and "How many in the room have ever experienced . . .?" If I suspect that anyone in the room could possibly be embarrassed by answering these questions, I preface my questions with statements such as the following. "I'd like to know a little about you in order to make sure that my lecture meets your needs. I'm going to ask a few questions and ask you to answer by raising your hands. So that no one need be concerned about the reactions of other people, will you all close your eyes for a minute while I ask questions and count hands." This action provides a measure of anonymity and security, and people are able to answer specific and rather personal questions without embarrassment.

Lecture Notes

In most methods of teaching it is possible to assess the learner's understanding of your material as you go along, to stop and clarify, to back up and explain, to correct a misstatement, and so on. When talking to one or two learners, or even a small group, this may not cause too much disruption, but during most lectures such clarification is not feasible, and so a confusing or disorganized lecture is likely to result in confused or disorganized learning of the material presented. It is essential, therefore, that your lecture be well organized, with good transitions between major ideas to make it easy for listeners to follow your train of thought. Otherwise, the listener is forced to play a kind of hide-and-seek with the nearly hidden main ideas. It may also help your listener if you number each of a series of points. The listener can follow your train of thought easily when he hears you say, "There are three points to consider. The first point is. . . . Point number two is . . .," and so on.

When preparing your lecture, try to avoid the phrase "as you all know" or "as everyone knows." Even if the phrase represents a cliché, not an assumption, it tends to alienate or irritate those listeners who do *not* know, and who may feel stupid when you imply that everyone else does.

Once you have developed your lecture, decide whether you want to speak from cards, pages of notes, or a copy of the complete lecture. Your preference is likely to change from occasion to occasion over the years; in the beginning it is important to use whichever system gives you the greatest security.

If you use a verbatim copy of your lecture, it should be typed and double spaced for easy reading. Underline headings and main divisions so that you can find your place easily. Rehearse and rehearse and rehearse, so that you are not completely dependent upon the typed page and can look up frequently and maintain at least minimal eye contact with your audience. Nothing is more deadly for an audience than having to sit and listen to a lecturer read a lengthy paper, head down, giving scarcely any indication of an awareness that an audience is present.

Notes or an outline will give you much greater flexibility than a copy of the complete text. With notes, it is easier to expand one point, to condense others, or to leave a few sections out completely in response to feedback from the audience. Such feedback may be nonverbal, but the cues are relatively easy to read. Restlessness, whispering, frequent changes of position, dozing or sleeping, and frequent glances at the wall clock are among the many observable cues of boredom and inattention that are likely to result from a dull or poorly organized lecture. (Should you ever encounter such a situation, don't panic! Quickly assess other possible causes. The room may be unbearably hot, and your lecture may be fine.) On the other hand, the absence of noise and movement, attentive postures, eyes focused on you, possibly some note taking, and a general feel of rapport indicate interest and attention.

It is a good idea to time your lecture. Modify it as needed until you are able to finish within five minutes of the allotted time. Lectures are commonly about an hour in length. If the lecture is described as a "talk," it is likely to be allotted from 20 to 60 minutes.

If you have access to a tape recorder, tape either a rehearsal or the actual lecture. Then, analyze the taped lecture for patterns of speech, inflection, tone, and volume. Was your voice interesting, or was it monotonous? Was each word carefully enunciated? How many times did you say "Uh"? Do you tend to introduce and punctuate each sentence with "OK?" or "Right?"? If you have access to a video tape recorder, you can analyze your gestures, mannerisms, posture, and facial expressions. If you cannot tape a rehearsal or the lecture, ask a friend to give you feedback that will help you present your material effectively.

Format and Plans for Presentation

First of all, decide whether or not there will be a time for questions. If so, how long? How will questions be submitted? Do you want questions to be written out and sent to the front of the room? Do you prefer to have each questioner stand and give his question aloud?

Are people likely to want to take notes? Will this distract you? If so, would it be possible to distribute a printed or dittoed outline at the beginning of your lecture in order to minimize the need for extensive note taking? If the material is sufficiently important, funds may be available that would allow you to distribute copies of your lecture, either free or for a small charge. Occasionally, an important address is published in a professional journal, and the audience can read it there. If you audiotape your lecture, you may want to make a copy available to people who missed the lecture, who want to review it, and so on.

Request, in advance, the equipment you will need. Don't assume that it will be available, no matter how simple or basic it may be. If there is no blackboard, request a portable one. If you feel uneasy about turning your back to the audience in order to write on the blackboard, request an overhead projector. This enables you to write on an acetate sheet while facing the audience, and to have the words or diagrams projected on a screen behind you, large enough for all to read.

If you have a soft voice and the acoustics in the room are poor, request a microphone. If there is no clock in the room, plan to wear a watch or bring a tiny clock. If you expect to be nervous and are worried that excessive hand movements may distract your listeners, try straightening and bending a paper clip as you talk. It provides an unobtrusive and acceptable outlet for excess nervous tension. Finally, you may want to request a glass of water, as the stress of anticipation may give you a dry mouth at the beginning of your lecture.

Presentation

Introduce yourself as needed, giving information about your background and your interest and involvement in the topic of your lecture.

Introduce the lecture. Describe briefly its topic, context, and scope. Tell the audience briefly what you are going to cover.

Describe the format. If there is to be a question-and-answer period, tell the audience at the beginning of the lecture so that they will be prepared to submit questions, either orally or in writing. Tell them about printed materials that will be available. If you are not using a microphone, ask whether everyone can hear you.

Give your lecture and watch the time. Read the cues from the audience as you go along. If you sense that you have lost their attention or that they are confused, that they are not with you, you may be able to modify the remaining material and recapture your rapport with the audience. You may, however, encounter an audience that is rather unresponsive. This phenomenon is disturbing, but it can happen in nursing just as easily as in show business.

Summarize at the end of the lecture or after a question-and-answer period. Briefly review what you have just said, using a slightly different approach. But if you expect the audience to stay and ask questions, don't sound as if you are dismissing them.

Repeat, or read aloud, each question before you answer it. An excellent answer teaches little unless the audience knows what the question is. You will need to take the initiative to end the questioning unless there is someone presiding over the session. Let the audience know, for example, when time is nearly up, or when there is time for only one more question.

GROUP DISCUSSION

Learning in a small group can be very different from learning in a large group, but not necessarily. The nature of the learning that occurs in a small group is not a function of the size of the group, but of the intent of the teacher. In some small groups there may be no discussion at all; the teacher talks to the learners and, in essence, gives a lecture to a small number of people. The learning that occurs is the same as if there had been 200 people in the room. In other settings there may be some discussion between teacher and students, but virtually no discussion between students. The learners are instructed as a group, but they are not taught by the group discussion method.

In a lecture, information is *acquired* as the teacher talks to the group. In group discussion, information is *used* as members of the group talk with each other. In a lecture, with some exceptions, much of the learning is the acquisition of new information, which will be used and applied at a later date. In group discussion, previously learned material, plus some new material, is applied and integrated, giving new insights and meanings and solutions to problems.

In a lecture, it is usually not feasible or possible to deal with personal feelings, values, reactions, and meanings. In group discussion, it is possible to explore meanings, examine values, and share feelings and reactions with each other. If the teacher is skilled and her intention is to focus primarily on people (rather than content), learning that occurs through group discussion will be highly personal, much different from the learning that results from group instruction or lecture. Neither type of teaching is best; the choice depends upon the type of learning that is needed in order to reach the desired objectives.

Purposes of Group Discussions

Some of the many reasons for using group discussion are:

- to motivate, stimulate, and create interest
- to seek action, effect change, promote new legislation or policy
- to share experiences and support each other.

Group discussion provides an opportunity for people to learn from each other, to learn from someone "who really knows," from someone with a similar problem, from someone who has found an answer. Examples of such groups would include persons who are terminally ill, spouses of patients with cardiac conditions, obese adolescents, parents of handicapped children, single parents, and so on.

Role and Functions of the Teacher

Prepare the environment. Arrive early and set up the room (or designate someone to do it). The setting should be informal, with people sitting in a circle or around a table. It is important that no one have his back to the others, unless the group is large enough (or the room small enough) to necessitate a double circle of chairs. In some situations, coffee helps people to relax and helps create a warm, informal atmosphere. The provision of adequate ashtrays, once a traditional part of preparations for a group meeting, is not now appropriate in light of current trends to protect the rights of nonsmokers.

Convene the group. You will know whether the group is meeting once only, with little or no chance of future contact, or whether sustained contact is likely, with group cohesiveness being a desired goal. Even if this is a once-only encounter, name tags or name cards at each person's place will help people address each other. If anonymity of group members is important, as in Overeaters Anonymous or in a group of current or potential child abusers, name tags giving first names only will still enable people to respond to each other in a personal way. The time spent on introductions is almost always worth while in establishing rapport between members, especially if each member describes in a sentence or two his current situation and his reason for being present.

Assess the group.   If this is a new group, note the age span and the basis or reason for the group. In all groups, assess the levels of stress, interest, and energy, determine whether attendance is voluntary or mandatory, and evaluate group comfort.

Establish norms.   Clarify expectations, describe the schedule, indicate scheduled breaks (have a watch available or designate someone to keep track of time), attend to any cultural or ethnic aspects, and bring new members up to date.

Facilitate discussion.   You may choose to initiate the discussion by presenting a predictable problem, something that your experience has shown to be common to many patients and families. You might present a hypothetical situation for discussion or merely state in general, "I have found that many patients experience. . . ." This approach may seem safer and less threatening to a new group than exposure of a personal situation or experience. In other situations you may stimulate discussion with questions such as, "What do you expect will happen if . . .?" and "What do you anticipate will be the hardest part of . . .?" When the members of the group feel safe and secure enough with each other, they will spontaneously introduce problems they have encountered, or report on developments in their situations since the group's last meeting.

Read the verbal and nonverbal cues as the discussion progresses. Encourage wide participation, but respect each person's right to remain silent and listen. Use caution in "calling on" a specific person—he may be deeply involved and unable to participate at the moment. Encourage persons to seek clarification and validation from each other, and to express empathy and concern *overtly.* Reinforce desired group behaviors. (Reinforcement is discussed in detail in Chapter 15). Refocus the group's attention and discussion when necessary. Use additional teaching techniques, such as role-playing, as indicated. Contribute, but don't lecture, preach, advise, or monopolize. Learn to tolerate silence. Force yourself to count to increasingly higher numbers before you break a period of silence, which may be extremely meaningful to those who are quietly thinking.

Evaluate the outcomes. In many respects, the outcomes of a group discussion are less predictable than the outcomes of any other method of teaching. The nature of the topics discussed, the flexibility of the situation, and the large amount of input from members of the group all contribute to varying outcomes.

Whenever feasible, it is desirable to have the group spend a few minutes evaluating the outcomes. A few questions, such as "What happened in our group today?" "What did you learn today?," or "In your opinion, what was the most important thing that we discussed today?," will usually help members of the group identify the significant aspects of the session. By comparing the group's responses with your objectives for the discussion, you will be able to estimate the effectiveness of the interactions.

You may want to make a few notes for future reference about the questions, techniques, or strategies that you found to be either effective or ineffective. The ability to lead a group discussion with confidence and expertise may not develop as easily or as quickly as you would like, but a careful analysis of each experience will speed the process of acquiring a skill that will be invaluable in many aspects of your professional life.

EXPLANATIONS

An explanation is perhaps the most frequently used (and abused) method of teaching. Properly used, an explanation is a response to the learner's need, real or potential. Misused, an explanation is likely to be involve one person's telling another person what he must do and why. The content of the explanation may be almost the same, but the approach and results are very different.

Teacher-Initiated Explanations

An explanation may be initiated by the teacher in anticipation of the learner's need or in response to a question. The teacher selects the content on the basis of:

- Past experience in similar situations
  Such an explanation is often prefaced by phrases such as "Many patients . . ." or "I have discovered that. . . ."

- Observations or assessments made in the present situation
  Such explanations usually state the assessment and the action to be taken, such as "Based on . . .,I am going to . . . ."
- Agency policy or protocol
  Examples of such explanations include visiting regulations, preoperative routines, agency policies, and the like.

Guidelines for Teacher-Initiated Explanations

Gain the learner's attention. Enhance motivation to learn by establishing a need. For example, don't launch into an explanation of how to cough, turn, and deep breathe (regardless of the patient's interest) and don't tell him what will happen if he doesn't do it. Instead, spend a few minutes describing the advantages of coughing, turning, and deep breathing, thereby making it a desirable activity. "After surgery, you will be able to . . . and will notice less . . . if you will cough, turn, and deep breath at frequent intervals. You will be uncomfortable as you do it at first, but your recovery will be so much smoother that you will be able to. . . ."

Give complete explanations. Give the details of who, what, where, when, why, and how, even to a child. The level and complexity of the explanation will vary from patient to patient, but the accuracy and completeness of basic information will not.

Assess the learner as you proceed. Assess his *knowledge.* He may have had three barium enemas before this one.

Assess his understanding. He may have had three barium enemas before this one but not understood what they were for or what was indicated by the results.

Assess his reaction. Look for verbal or nonverbal indications of relief, confusion, increased stress, interest, and so on and adjust your explanation accordingly.

Explanations Given in Response to a Question

The question's format and wording may give you some clues to its meaning to the patient. Questions that ask Who? What? Where? When? and How? are often simple requests for information, although often the person is expressing his underlying fear, worry, anger, or other emotion through his questions. An explanation is useful if the patient is seeking information; it is of little use if the patient is expressing his feelings.

A question that begins with Why? usually asks the purpose, rationale, reason, or basis for a decision or action. It usually involves values and beliefs and may have a high emotional component. It is important to listen for the underlying concern of such questions as, "Why do I have to . . .?," "Why does the doctor . . .?," and "Why do you always . . .?" It is very easy to become defensive and offer explanations to justify the behavior of yourself or the staff, when in reality the patient may be asking, "Are these things happening because I am critically ill?" or "Are you really competent?" If this is the case, an explanation of your behavior is not likely to be as helpful as a discussion of his fears would be.

Guidelines for Explanations in Response to Questions

1. *Take your time.* Make sure that you understand both the question and what it means to the patient. Clarify your understanding of the question, rephrase it, and validate your perception. Sometimes you may want to answer the question briefly, then take time to determine the patient's reason for asking it.

2. *Initially, don't give more information than was asked for.* If your answer is satisfying, he will feel free to ask another question. You have heard the phrase "hungry for information." Using that metaphor, I would say that "If he's still hungry, he'll ask for seconds" and "If the first taste was good, he'll ask for more." You have probably had the experience of asking someone a question, expecting a one- or two-sentence response, and receiving instead such a long and detailed answer that you wished you had never asked. You may have learned little except not to ask that person anything again.

In some situations, however, you may choose to end your explanation with a bit of information or a question to stimulate the learner, to whet his curiosity, to give him something to think about and provide the basis for more questions.

3. *Ask for feedback—be direct.* Before you leave the patient, or before the subject is changed, ask the patient questions such as "Does that answer your question?," "Does that help to clear it up for you?," or "Is there anything else I might be able to explain to you?"

4. *Look for nonverbal feedback.* Watch for cues that might indicate understanding or the lack of it, such as a gaze of bewilderment, a nod of understanding, or a look of puzzlement. Verbalize these observations to the patient, and on the basis of his response, modify or expand your explanation as needed.

5. *If you can't explain, be honest.* Don't be curt or evasive. An honest response, such as "I don't know, but I'll try to find out," "I can't talk just now, because I'm . . .," or "I'm concentrating on . . . now; I'll be able to answer in just a moment," conveys interest and encourages future questions.

EXPLORATION

Exploration is rarely listed as a separate teaching strategy. It is often considered as one aspect of other techniques such as discussion, role-playing, or discovery. I believe that it merits separate attention, especially with respect to patient teaching and health education.

Patient teaching is often viewed as leading to the acquisition of more knowledge, facts, data, and information. In many situations a more appropriate goal would be the acquisition of an increased ability to use existing knowledge. The patient may have no need for more data, but rather a need for an increased ability to analyze and synthesize existing data, to make sense of what he has learned. He may be feeling overwhelmed by his experiences, bewildered by his situation, and confused by ambivalent feelings. Additional information does not add to his comfort—it adds to his problem, because now he has even more information to cope with.

Teaching through exploration is one of the most difficult of all teaching strategies, because it requires great restraint to keep from giving more information, offering advice, and providing detailed explanations. These behaviors reflect a natural tendency to want to help by giving an answer, by providing a solution for the troubled person. In most situations, however, there are no answers that can be "given" to the person, no solutions that can be "handed" to him.

Teaching by exploration is based on a belief that answers to problems come from the learner himself, that solutions lie within the person who is experiencing the difficulty. The role of the teacher is to help the person examine the situation and/or his feelings about it, to identify possible responses or courses of action and to consider their likely consequences. For example, as you help Mrs. Smith prepare for her mother's discharge from the hospital, you notice that she becomes very upset as she tries to decide which first-floor room to convert to a temporary bedroom. You realize that she does not need further information regarding the relative merits of various rooms, or possible placement of furniture, or the importance of access to the bathroom.

You have reason to believe that she needs to explore her fear of the reaction of her teenage children and her husband to the disruption in living arrangements. Mrs. Smith may need to examine her relationship to her mother and the relationships within the family. She may need help in assessing the impact of such a move on the family and in considering possible alternative courses of action. As you and the patient explore the situation together, Mrs. Smith gains new insights, a fresh perspective, and a different outlook. After exploring the issue with you, she is likely to be motivated to learn whatever is needed to resolve the problem. She might, for example, decide that she needs to learn to be more assertive. If so, that may be what she needs to learn, not how to rearrange rooms.

Teaching through exploration requires an intense application of basic communication skills. No unusual or extraordinary skills are needed, but the teaching behaviors listed below presume that basic interpersonal skills are part of your repertoire of nursing interactions.

The nurse who is helping a patient learn through the process of exploring an issue or problem will exhibit the following behaviors. She will:

1. listen carefully
2. encourage the patient to express his feelings
3. help the patient to examine all possible aspects of the situation
4. use questions judiciously, cautiously, and carefully (as if questions were limited and in short supply!)
5. clarify her own perceptions of the situation
6. share her own perceptions with the patient
7. confront the patient with seeming discrepancies between verbal and nonverbal cues
8. help patient discover relationships between ideas and values
9. convey empathy and concern.
10. refrain from giving advice or additional information until a desired behavior or course of action is chosen by the patient and specific help is requested.

To summarize, exploration is a method of teaching that helps the patient or family member to:

• recall and integrate previous learning
• learn problem-solving skills

- explore the meaning of abstract concepts such as suffering, pain, or death and dying
- clarify values and beliefs.

A common outcome of exploration is a period of consolidation and integration of previous learning, a time of pulling things together. This is often followed by the learner's recognition of the need for additional information, greater knowledge, or new skills, which produces a corresponding increase in motivation to learn.

DEMONSTRATION

Demonstrations range in complexity and scope along a continuum from a spontaneous "Here, let me show you" through a planned, more formal demonstration to a completely planned, rehearsed, and filmed demonstration in which even the narration is scripted, word for word, and synchronized with the action. A spontaneous, spur-of-the-moment demonstration is neither better nor worse than a carefully planned and executed one; the choice depends upon the situation. You can't afford to miss an opportunity for teaching by delaying until you have had time to plan a demonstration, but neither can you afford to give a formal demonstration with the casual approach of a spontaneous one.

All demonstrations share certain characteristics. Let us look briefly at the special aspects of a spontaneous demonstration and then examine demonstrations in general.

Spontaneous Demonstrations

Spontaneous demonstration is a nursing intervention that responds to a person's need to learn how to do something at once. You may notice the person's frustration over being unable to complete a task, or he may ask for help in doing something. You may realize that a critical bit of teaching had been omitted on the previous home visit, or that the patient is being discharged earlier than expected. A new and urgent need may have suddenly arisen as a result of a change in the patient's condition or situation.

When you sense that you may need to demonstrate a skill or task for a person who is struggling to do something, the first step is: Wait a minute. Don't rush in too fast. A careful assessment of the situation, of the person's intent, of his need and his desire for help may indicate that a demonstration is not required. He may need support, recognition of his progress so far, and encouragement to persevere a bit longer. He may act completely frustrated, but not yet be willing to accept help.

If a demonstration is warranted, show him what is currently needed. Then, plan an appropriate follow-up rather than overwhelming him with more than he can handle at the moment. A spur-of-the-moment demonstration may involve a sense of urgency that makes it difficult for the learner to absorb as much as he might in a less hurried situation. If you are not able to do the follow-up teaching yourself, describe the need for additional teaching in your referral to another agency.

Finally, even though you may be responding rather quickly to a person's need to learn, so that you have little time for planning, use as many techniques and actions of a planned demonstration as are possible and appropriate.

Planned Demonstration

A planned demonstration is used to help the patient acquire a skill that will enable him to maintain his own health, participate in his own care, and care for himself or others. The skill may be manual or interpersonal. The demonstration of a manual skill, when followed by a practice session, effectively combines the learning that occurs through hearing, seeing, touch, and manipulation. (Demonstrations designed to teach interpersonal skills are described in later sections on role modeling and role playing.) A demonstration may also be used to orient a person to a procedure or process. You may demonstrate, in advance, a treatment that the patient will soon experience, or you may show him what will happen during a forthcoming procedure. If a person can see and handle any equipment that will be used, he will learn much more than if he is merely told about it. Such demonstrations may be given to an individual patient or to a group.

Preparation for a Demonstration

Preparation of self. Practice both the demonstration and the verbal explanation as needed. Decide where you will place equipment, how you will dispose of waste materials, when containers should be opened, and so on. It is most disconcerting to find oneself in the middle of an otherwise smooth demonstration with both hands full, and the cover not yet unscrewed on the next piece of equipment to be used.

Assemble the equipment and do the demonstration or procedure in the way it will be experienced or used by the patient. Modifications can be made later, but it is too confusing to the patient to be taught: "This is the way it is usually done. Learn this and then you can learn the way you will do it." If necessary, delay the demonstration until the actual equipment to be used is available, until you can visit the patient's home, or until you can do whatever must be done in order for the demonstration to be relevant to the persons involved.

As you rehearse, try to anticipate possible reactions of the learners. Based on your own past experience, has this particular skill seemed interesting, frightening, or difficult to learn? Based upon your assessment of the current learners, are they likely to be interested, bored, or overwhelmed? Any prediction you can make is likely to be useful in your preparation.

Preparation of patient. Preparation of the patient will be based upon your assessments and the plans that have been made. Create interest and get attention, based on his needs. Whenever possible, set a time with the patient for the demonstration. Describe the demonstration's purpose and intent. Tell where it will be held and who will be there. Describe the probable benefits, based upon the patient's needs and motivation.

Occasionally, you may be caring for a patient or family who cannot tolerate extensive preparation or formal instruction. In such a situation, you will need to integrate any demonstrations into other nursing interventions, showing him in a seemingly casual way how to do only one aspect of the necessary skill at any one time. Such partial or mini demonstrations, which might appear spontaneous, will be as carefully planned as a more extensive, complete demonstration.

Planning the demonstration. Given as much information as possible about the learner(s), you will need to consider a number of factors in planning a demonstration. Some of the most important are listed below, with no significance attached to the order.

1. Is there an optimal angle for viewing? If the skill that the learner is expected to duplicate requires fine motor skills, he may need to view the demonstration while looking over your shoulder in order to see it as he will do it. If he watches the demonstration while sitting facing you, he will need to mentally reverse each action before he can duplicate it. If the group is small, a few people can stand beside you or behind you. If the group is large, you may need to use a video tape that you have made, or a commercially prepared filmstrip or slides taken from an over-the-shoulder angle.

2. How will you phrase the rationale, the reason for each action? Depending upon the characteristics of the learners, will you teach by rote memorization, or by inquiry, or by some approach midway

between the two? For example, will you teach *THE* way to do the task, will you teach *ONE* of many ways, or will you help the learner to devise *A* way to accomplish the task? A child, a very anxious person, or a retarded person will probably learn more effectively from a simple, direct, structured approach that says, "This is the way to do it." With this approach, there is no confusion or ambiguity. An intelligent adolescent, however, may do better with an introductory demonstration, followed by an exploration of "What would be the best way for you to accomplish the same thing?" When using the latter approach, you will need a) to be open to a variety of answers from learners, some of which may seem very unorthodox, and b) to thoroughly understand the underlying principles of chemistry, physics, microbiology, physiology, or whatever is needed to evaluate the safety and effectiveness of the learner's desired method of doing the task.

In any event, you must let the learner know whether he is to follow the demonstration exactly or whether you will help him devise a personalized version. An example of these different approaches can be seen in teaching a new mother the simple requirement that she have clean hands before starting to bathe her newborn infant or make formula. One person might be able to base her actions upon her current situation. If she had just finished cleaning the cat's litter box, she would obviously scrub her hands thoroughly. If she had just finished washing dishes in hot soapy water, she could safely assume that her hands were clean. On the other hand, a person who learned slowly might function more effectively if she learned that "you always wash your hands for a full minute before handling the baby or making formula." A careful assessment of the learner will help you decide upon the apporach to be used. The point is, no one set of explanations is appropriate for all learners.

3. How will you make the transition from your initial demonstration to a satisfactory return demonstration by the patients? In some situations, it will be feasible for you to demonstrate an activity, and for the learner to repeat the demonstration at once. In many other situations, the first and last demonstrations will be separated by a number of others, characterized by a gradual decrease of participation on your part and a gradual increase in patient participation. This process will be accompanied by fewer and fewer verbal cues from you. For example:

Demonstration 1:   You do the task while describing your actions and rationale

Demonstration 2:   You do the task while the patient describes in his own words what you are doing, or

Demonstration 3:   The patient does the task while you "talk him through it."(The patient may prefer to reverse the order of demonstrations 2 and 3 or may feel that they can be omitted.)

Demonstration 4:   (With or without the benefit of practice sessions, depending upon the patient)
The patient does the task and describes his actions and the rationale for each.
The patient may give a single return demonstration, or it may be a gradual process over a period of time, with the patient doing more of the task each day. You may encourage and help the patient as you say, "You hold . . . while I . . .," or "I'll do . . . while you. . . ."

The number of demonstrations will depend upon the capability of the learner, the type of complexity of the skill to be acquired, and the level of competency needed by the learner.

Giving the Demonstration

When the learners have assembled, make certain that every one can see your demonstration. Take time to rearrange chairs, encourage people to move closer, do whatever is necessary so that everyone will have a unobstructed view of the demonstration.

Give a brief introduction.   Explain what is to be learned, what use can be made of the learning, and what should be observed or noted.

Begin the demonstration.   Whenever possible, run through the procedure or demonstration rather quickly to given an overview and enable the learners to get a sense of what is to be learned. Be sure to mention that a slower, more detailed demonstration will follow.

Demonstrate again.   Make clear to the learners whether this is THE way to do it (for example, how to keep an object sterile) or whether this one of many ways to do it. Expand your explanation, giving a more complete rationale for each action than you did the first time.

If the task is complex or anxiety-producing, try to repeat the demonstration a third time. This time direct the learners to interrupt you as needed, and encourage them to ask questions.

Arrange for practice as needed, either now or later. If the task involves sterile technique, it is usually helpful to let the learners handle the unsterile equipment until they are thoroughly familiar with it. For example, let the diabetic patient manipulate and unsterile syringe and needle and get the "feel" of it. The need to be dexterous with a sterile one places a double burden on him—learning to maintain sterility while learning to manipulate a syringe. In other situations, analyze the skill to determine its component parts, and then make provision for the patient to learn them one at a time rather than several at once.

Arrange for a return demonstration. Assess the learner's performance and evaluate his skill. Evaluate his understanding by assessing his ability to recognize his own errors and his ability to correct errors that you point out. Based on learner performance, make plans to do supplemental teaching as needed, changing method or pacing as indicated to help the learner acquire the skill. Plan practice sessions as needed.

Insure transfer of learning. Help the learner anticipate the possible problems and reasonable solutions. Ask him "What would you do if . . .?" and help him work through any problems that he might encounter. If he is in a hospital, ask him to have his own equipment brought in to him so he can practice with it before discharge. Discuss the maintenance of equipment, purchase of replacement parts, possible substitutes in an emergency, and so on with him as soon as he is thoroughly comfortable with the task. Give him printed materials, if available, for review at a later date or to supplement your teaching.

Filmed and Taped Demonstrations

In a number of situations it would be well to consider filming or videotaping your demonstration. Some of these situations are:

- when direct observation is not possible and a simulated demonstration is not feasible. For example, it is usually not possible for a patient to observe a cardiac catheterization, and it is not possible to orient him to the procedure by a simulated demonstration, but you might be able to make a video tape of the procedure, which could then be used in the orientation of many patients who are to undergo it.
- when the demonstration is given frequently to rather large groups who find it difficult to get close enough to see well. A film or video

tape makes it possible to project a close-up view, taken from any angle, to the entire group.

- when a given teacher has perfected an effective demonstration of a difficult task, and is willing to share her expertise with other nurses by letting them show the film or tape to their patients.
- when a given demonstration is infrequently needed, but is sufficiently important that it must be given whenever it is needed, sometimes on rather short notice and with no one ready to give it.

The use of a videotaped demonstration insures that the instruction of various groups will be uniform and consistent and still permits the nurse to modify the presentation with additional examples or discussion to meet the needs of the group.

ROLE PLAYING

Role playing occupies a unique place among teaching methods and strategies. On one hand, it seems simple and spontaneous, very much like the "let's pretend" of childhood: "You be the princess and I'll be the wicked stepmother" or "You be the mother and I'll be the father. . . ." On the other hand, it is a complex and powerful way to facilitate learning. Role playing may be described as a brief, usually spontaneous interaction in which several persons play out roles that are assigned, but unrehearsed. Both the players and the rest of the class usually become deeply involved.

Role playing provides an opportunity for learners to:

1. explore alternative ways of acting or responding in a situation.
2. see how others might do it, hear how various responses sound, and see how other people might respond or react.
3. practice a new behavior in a safe and supportive setting.

Role playing may be used to promote involvement in a situation, to evoke an emotional response, to give a common basis for discussion, to focus a generalized or diffuse discussion.

You may resort to role playing infrequently, but when you do use it, the effect can be almost magical. It can be like a trump card, a free turn, or an ace up your sleeve.

The cues for using role playing are often subtle and easily missed. If, however, you decide to include it in your repertoire of teaching techniques, you will find opportunities to use it with increasing frequency. You will become aware of patient comments or statements that suggest a need for working through a situation or problem. For example, "I don't think I could do that" or "I could never do that" often indicates a need to test out a new behavior or to prepare for a future event. Role playing gives the person an opportunity to act out and cope with the fantasy that emerges as people discuss the question, "What's the worst thing that could possibly happen if you . . . .?" Role playing gives an opportunity to plan ahead, to be prepared with several possible responses to "the worst thing that could possibly happen." It gives a learner a chance to figure ways to handle a variety of possible responses to possible reactions of others.

An argument, confrontation, or stalemate in a discussion might lead you to speculate aloud: "I wonder what would happen if . . .?" and to follow up with a role playing situation. You might be very direct and say, "Let's role-play this situation and see what happens," if you believe the learners have had experience with role playing and will be comfortable doing so. If you feel that role playing may be new or strange, as it well might be to a group of senior citizens, for example, you might be less direct. Instead of referring to role playing as such, you could say, "Let's see what might happen in a hypothetical (or imaginary) situation. Let's imagine that. . . ." With children, the age-old invitation "Let's pretend that . . ." is as irresistible as ever.

Guidelines for Role Playing

The first step in role playing is to describe the situation briefly. You might use the situation under discussion, unless you feel it might be embarrassing or threatening to the patient or family member who brought it up. It may seem safer if you describe a hypothetical situation similar to the one that prompted the role playing.

Next, describe the roles, giving age, sex, and relationships of players, and ask for volunteers. In almost every situation, someone will volunteer for each role. It may be the most unlikely person—there is a certain safety in playing the role of someone else and it provides a chance to do or say things you would never do in real life. In the rare instances in which you do not have enough volunteers, it is important to remember that, as a rule, you never assign a role to a person who exemplifies or typifies the role to be played. Otherwise, during the discussion that follows role playing, it will be hard to separate the role from the real person, and the player may feel that the others are talking about *him* rather than the role he was playing.

Once players have been designated, give any necessary directions. Very few are needed and they are usually given to all players, within earshot of everyone. On occasion, you may need or want to give a few separate directions. For example, you might want to tell the "parent": "If the 'child' acts angry, respond as suggested by Dr. Ginott—so we can ask him how it felt when you did so." Have the players move close together. No props are needed and there is no script, of course. You may want to briefly clarify or review the purpose and intent of the role playing, and tell the group what to look for.

Stop the action after five to 10 minutes, sometimes less, rarely more. Stop the action at a logical pause, at the conclusion of a specific interaction, as soon as any conflict seems to be resolved, and while interest is high. Don't let the role playing die and the action peter out, because attention and interest will drop and the desired involvement of learners will cease.

Make use of the role-playing experience. Much learning occurs in the period immediately after role playing, especially if the teacher follows the suggestions listed below.

1. Ask each player to describe his feelings—they may or may not have been expressed freely or accurately in words during the role playing. The audience needs to hear such comments as "I was furious, but I didn't feel I had a right to . . .," or "I felt so scared of her that I couldn't think of anything to say."
2. Ask the audience to describe their feelings about the interaction and the feelings that the scene evoked. For example, a member of the audience might say, "I felt like I did when I first heard that Carrie had leukemia." It is important not to rush; this period may give a person an opportunity to express feelings that up until now have been difficult to verbalize.

Finally, help the group to learn from the role playing. The function of the teacher is to:

• help the learners to analyze the action, to discover reasons why people might respond or behave in such a way
• suggest alternative actions
• hypothesize about the possible effects or outcomes of various suggested behaviors
• possibly test out a likely approach or solution through a second bit of role playing.

Many teachers find that it takes a fair amount of self-confidence to use role playing. This confidence can be developed in three ways.

1. Practice and rehearse mentally. Look for opportunities to role-play; plan what you would do. Anticipate the worst thing that could happen (usually nothing worse than an open expression of boredom by the learners) and mentally explore possible reactions and responses. Once you have rehearsed this a few times, it will not seem strange and new to hear yourself actually saying aloud, "Let's role-play it and find out."
2. Practice "let's pretend" with children. They are likely to be eager and noncritical. You will be able to initiate role playing in a nonthreatening situation. (Of course, if children make you more nervous than role playing does, omit this suggestion and try the next one.)
3. Suggest mini-role plays in noncritical situations. During the course of ordinary conversations, explore an idea by asking, "What would you say to me if you were . . . and I said . . .?" A spouse, neighbor, child, or friend will probably answer you, at which point you may feel that you can respond as if you were role playing.

Each bit of practice will help you to feel more comfortable with role playing and more confident in the use of this very effective teaching technique.

ROLE MODELING

Role modeling is based on social learning theory and is closely related to the processes of imitation and identification. Whereas in role playing you are "being someone else," in role modeling you are being yourself.

A role model is a person who demonstrates certain behaviors in a real-life setting. A mother provides her small daughter with a model of a woman's role in society. A nurse, interacting with a child, provides the mother with a model of effective mothering behaviors. A former patient may provide another patient with a model of acceptance and rehabilitation. The nurse's interaction with a physician can provide a model of assertive questioning for the patient who is reluctant to ask questions of that physician. In short, a role model provides a pattern, something to copy, in the area of interpersonal relationships.

Three conditions favor role modeling.

1. The behavior to be learned must be seen as desirable by the learner. Research in the area of social learning theory indicates that people will not imitate behavior that they perceive as eliciting negative or undesirable effects. The learner must experience a vicarious reward as he watches the role model. If the behavior results in enjoyment, satisfaction, or reward for the role model, the learner is likely to attempt to imitate that behavior.

   Therefore, if you are using role modeling as a teaching method, it is important for you to make sure that the learner is fully aware of all desirable outcomes. Sometimes the outcomes are obvious. The mobility and agility of a rehabilitated patient may speak for the effort previously expended by that patient. Sometimes the outcome needs to be pointed out. You may need to verbalize the satisfaction you receive in order to help the learner see the behavior as desirable. Statements such as "It always makes me feel better when I am able to . . ." or "It makes my day go better when I . . ." are likely to foster a positive attitude toward the observed behavior. Anything you can do that helps the learner view the behavior as desirable will increase the likelihood that he will copy that behavior.

2. The learner must be capable of copying the behavior that he observes. If he is intellectually, physically, or emotionally incapable of duplicating the behavior of the role model, that behavior cannot be learned, no matter how desirable it may seem. Language difficulties, unmet safety and security needs, low self-esteem, depression, and mental retardation are but a few of the barriers to purposeful learning through imitation and identification.

3. The learner must know what to observe. The role model (or another person who may be directing the learning) must point out the essential cues to the learner. Unless he knows what to watch for, he may focus his attention on an interesting but peripheral aspect of the situation. You may have intended to role-model for a family an effective way to discuss a sensitive issue with an aging parent, but the family missed the role modeling because they were listening only to the details of the conversation itself. They may be able to recall some of your interaction IF you discuss the interactions with them immediately upon leaving the parent's room, but the role modeling would have been more effective had you indicated what they were to observe. You might have told them, before entering the room, "I'm going to try this approach today. I plan to say . . ., and

then if your mother says . . ., I will know that it is working and I'll proceed to. . . . You watch and tell me afterward how effective you think such an approach might be in the future."

Areas related to patient teaching in which role modeling is likely to be effective include parenting, communication skills, discipline, mental health, sex education, and interaction with terminally ill relatives. Regardless of the area, it is imperative that your role modeling be consistent with your usual behavior. If it is not, you are *assuming* a role. If you are a smoker, you cannot role-model nonsmoking behaviors. If you are by nature shy or lacking in self-confidence, you are not ready to role-model assertive behaviors. But given a role that is part of your repertoire of behavior and if attending to the three conditions described above, you will find role modeling an effective way to facilitate learning.

15

Use of Audiovisual Materials

Since materials that help her reach the learner through his ears and eyes provide audiovisual assistance, almost everything a teacher uses could be considered an AV aid. A book, a film, the label from a bottle, a TV documentary, or a patient's rash—all of these are audio, visual, or both. More specifically, however, the term designates instructional materials in the form of film, tape, television, radio, records, and some printed materials.

AUDIOVISUAL POSSIBILITIES

Audiovisual materials extend the teacher's capabilities and enrich the student's learning by removing barriers of time, space, accessibility, and the limitations of the human body. AV technology makes it possible to:

- capture experiences on tape or film, so that they are not forgotten but may be relived or experienced time and again by many people.
- transcend time and space and bring input from special people to the learner across thousands of miles. It might not be possible, in terms of time and money, to actually bring a famous physician or extraordinary patient to a discussion group or for a lecture in a small town, but an audiovisual presentation enables the learners to see and hear that special person, rather than just reading about him.
- take the learner to inaccessible places such as the delivery room, a research lab, a special patient's home, or a hospice in England.
- enable the learner to see things not visible to the naked eye and to hear sounds inaudible to the unaided ear, such as the division of a cell, the pattern of brain waves, and the sound of a fetal heart.
- enable the learner to watch procedures that cannot be simulated, such as lumbar puncture, cardiac catheterization, renal dialysis, or hyperalimentation.

150

- permit the learner to stop and examine a procedure or event, to back up, move ahead, repeat, skip segments, speed up the action—to do whatever is necessary in order to clearly understand and comprehend.
- give the learner the advantage of many modes of presentation. For example, a film may include models of real objects, pictures, diagrams, special sound and visual effects, human action, animation, and more.

USE OF AUDIOVISUAL RESOURCES

Since audiovisual materials have the potential for facilitating and enhancing learning, it is important to consider how they might be used to improve patient teaching. Some possible uses of audiovisual materials are:

- to stimulate learning, create interest, and motivate.
- to present essential content and information.
- to demonstrate a procedure to a large group.
- to orient patients to a ward, clinic, agency, or the like.
- to permit patients and families to make use of otherwise idle time, such as time spent in a waiting room.
- to permit successive persons or groups of persons to view a demonstration without endless repetition by the nurse.
- to permit the patient to control certain aspects of his own learning, such as pacing, review, amount of repetition, and the selection of mode of presentation.

Sometimes AV materials are essential, sometimes superfluous. If used when they are not needed, they are expensive, they may waste time, and in extreme situations they may actually interfere with learning by overloading the learner with too many stimuli.

Two fundamental questions to be asked are: "What are you trying to accomplish?" and "What help do you need?" Suppose that your objective is to help a patient understand how a laminectomy may reduce pain caused by a herniated disc. If the patient is an intern, a physical education major, or a nurse, a verbal explanation may suffice, because the patient understands the vocabulary as well as the anatomy and physiology of the spinal column and nervous system.

If the patient is an ophthalmologist who once knew, but has forgotten, the details of the relevant anatomy and physiology over the years, a simple sketch will refresh his memory. If you are talented, a pad of paper and pencil may yield all the AV assistance you will need in a majority of teaching situations.

If the patient is a person with no knowledge of his body, you may need diagrams or photographs of X-rays. If the patient has a limited ability to deal with relatively abstract concepts, you may need a few segments of vertebrae or a model of the spinal column.

SELECTION OF AUDIOVISUAL AIDS

Different levels of learning and different objectives in patient teaching and health education require different AV aids. These AV materials are used to supplement and complement your teaching; their use is never an end in itself. So, decide what you are trying to accomplish, what things you are unable to do without help, and what specific help AV materials could give you. Then, determine which AV aids could help you best.

In trying to determine what kind of audiovisual aids would enhance your teaching, ask yourself the following questions:

1. Do you need audio assistance? If so, why? What kind of audio help do you need?
2. Do you need visual assistance? Why? What kind is needed?
   a) Do you need color? Why? How will it help?
   b) Do you need motion? Why?
3. Do you need tactile stimuli, something for the learner to touch, hold, manipulate? If so, what kind of object? Why?

Notice the WHY? in each of these questions. It is important to use AV aids when they are *essential*; it is equally important to teach without them if they are peripheral or marginally useful. All AV materials cost money. Excessive or unnecessary use of these materials will increase the cost of health care without necessarily increasing its quality. Even if you save money by preparing some of your own materials, you have used time and energy that might have been spent on other professional activities. I am not *against* the use of AV materials. I am wholeheartedly in favor of audiovisual materials IF their use will truly help your patient to learn. I *am* against using AV aids simply because your agency has budgeted a certain sum for their purchase, or because "everybody seems to say that AV materials improve teaching," or because their use seems to bolster your confidence.

The following sections will explain some advantages and disadvantages of various types of AV softwear. (The term *software* refers to the materials, such as film, records, or tape, that carry the actual message; *hardware* refers to the equipment, such as the projector, that transmits this message.)

It is beyond the scope of this book to discuss all useful AV aids. Therefore, only the following will be included: audiotapes, videotapes, slides, filmstrips, motion pictures, film loops, and books.

Audiotapes

An autiotape is an excellent way to enhance learning when the patient does not need to see something in order to learn. For example, he might listen to a tape that reviews or expands the explanations given him by his physician, a tape of an interview with another patient who has coped successfully with a similar condition, a tape that suggests ways to explain a given diagnosis to one's children, or a tape telling a health-related story to children.

Audiotapes may be purchased from a publisher of educational materials, prepared by the AV department of your agency, or made with your own tape recorder. They are usually used in cassette form. Cassettes are easy to store and there is no danger of dropping a reel and having it unwind.

If you plan to make your own tapes, the following suggestions may help.

1. Practice with trivia until you have overcome any self-consciousness and mike fright. Try reading your professional journals into the mike as you experiment with control settings, voice levels, mike positions, and so on. (You will get your reading done and, at the same time, learn to feel comfortable while recording.) To get the feel of speaking without notes, recite poetry or nursery rhymes, or record imaginary conversations. Listen to your recorded voice for patterns of speech that might be distracting to a listener. Count the number of times you say "Okay," "Uh," or "Right." Listen for times when you mumble or drop your voice too low. As soon as you feel relatively comfortable and relaxed while recording, you are ready to make your tapes.

2. Whenever possible, use a reel-to-reel recorder for the initial recording of important or permanent tapes. The tape in a cassette is usually inaccessible for editing. Even a professional narrator occasionally misspeaks himself or mispronounces a word, and you are likely to

do so too. With a simple splicing kit (costing about $5) you can cut out the unacceptable section of tape and insert another section that you have recorded for that purpose. With a few hours practice, you will be able to delete phrases and even single words. When you have edited the tape to your satisfaction, you can re-record it on a cassette yourself, send it to a studio to have it done professionally, or possibly have the original edited tape placed into a cassette.

3. If you tape an interview with a patient, obtain his written permission to use the tape as a teaching aid. Conceivably he might say later that he did not give you permission to share the tape with anyone, that he did not understand what he was doing, that he was coerced. It is not likely, but it might happen. Or you might want to quote the patient in some article or book in the future, when you might be unable to locate the patient to get his permission. Check with your agency to see if they use a standard permission slip. Some agencies require that a duplicate permission slip be attached to the patient's chart or record. If there is no standard permission form, you will need to devise your own form and keep a copy for your own records. The essential elements are: date, patient's name, the activity for which permission is given, the purposes for which the product (photograph, tape, film, or whatever is to be used, patient's signature, and your signature. In some situations you may need to guarantee anonymity.

Videotape

If you plan to use television as a teaching aid, you will probably use recorded videotapes rather than live broadcasts. Videotapes can be purchased from a commercial producer, but they may or may not meet the needs of your teaching situation. Therefore, if you have access to a video tape recorder, by all means learn to use it. It is no more difficult to operate than an audio tape recorder—the tape deck is very similar to a reel-to-reel tape recorder. The camera is easy to focus and operate and, since many agencies have portable recording systems, you have the potential for creating a wide variety of educational materials for use in situations that require both sound and motion. You could videotape a demonstration for the use of nurses on other units, or to avoid repetition on your own unit. You could videotape a patient who has adapted well to a given condition—for example, a patient who has had a mastectomy, especially if there is no Reach to Recovery program in the area.

Try taking a lesson from physical education programs, in which the athlete is shown videotapes of himself so that he can analyze his actions in order to improve them. You can videotape a patient who is learning to walk with crutches or a new prosthesis in order to give him feedback about his performance and progress to date.

Children generally have a positive attitude toward television, and as videotape cassettes become more common and more inexpensive, television may become the medium of choice for pediatric patient teaching and health education.

If your agency has an audiovisual department, one of the technicians or staff may make the videotapes for you, once you have identified and outlined the content and described the necessary action. Compared to audiotapes, videotapes are relatively expensive, but by comparison with other media that might be used to show motion, videotape is inexpensive because it can be erased and reused.

Slides and Filmstrips

Slides and filmstrips are commonly used in conjunction with an audiotape or phonograph record, giving the learner a sharp, colored image accompanied by synchronized narration.

The images projected from slides and filmstrips are identical, but the cost, ease of handling, and equipment needed for projection are different. Slides require more storage space than the equivalent number of frames in a filmstrip. Slides are more expensive than filmstrips to prepare, because each frame must be individually mounted. Slides offer many advantages, however, which often outweigh the slightly higher cost.

Slides are not easily scratched because they are stored and projected from the same tray. Filmstrips are easily scratched because they are handled each time they are used; therefore, you might consider cutting your filmstrip into frames and mounting each frame as a slide. These new slides (frames of the filmstrip) can then be rearranged; the presentation can be shortened by deletion of some frames, or expanded by adding slides from a different source to meet your specific teaching needs.

Slides offer great flexibility in teaching because:

1. They are easy to rearrange if a different sequence is desired.
2. You can update a group of slides by adding slides or replacing those that are outdated with more current ones.
3. You can upgrade a slide presentation over a period of time by gradually replacing single slides with ones of better quality as they become available.

4. Since it is relatively inexpensive to duplicate slides, it is feasible to develop a number of programs using portions of a single set of slides and different tapes; for example, you could:
   - use a full set of 40 slides plus tape 1 for a newly diagnosed patient.
   - use slides 1, 2, 8, 13, and 25–40 with tape 2 for teaching self-care.
   - use slides 1, 2, 8, 13, 19, 25, 28, 31, 37, and 40 with tape 3 for review.
   - use slides 1, 2, 8, 13, 19, 25, 28, 31, 37, and 40 with tape 4 for testing and evaluation.

If you want to develop your own slide presentation, find out if your agency has a photographer on its staff who might take the slides for you. If not, you can do your own photography. Most cameras, even inexpensive Kodak Instamatics, will take slides, and with a bit of expertise and some good books on the subject you can easily prepare an effective set of slides. Most commercial slides and filmstrips are synchronized with a record or cassette tape. A local AV studio can synchronize your slides with your own audiotape.

You could prepare a series of slide-tape presentations on a variety of topics for the use of patients in the waiting rooms of clinics, or for families who spend long hours in waiting rooms outside intensive care units or while waiting for patients in surgery. A presentation in the admitting office could orient the patient and his family to the hospital. Since a tray of slides, a slide projector, and a cassette tape player are relatively easy to carry, you could take slide-tape programs (or filmstrip-tape programs) to the patient's home to help teach him and/or his family.

16mm Films

Sixteen-millimeter films are perhaps the most familiar of all audiovisual media. They are the standard movies shown in classrooms across the country. Because 16mm films are expensive, most agencies and institutions do not buy them but rather borrow or rent them from a film library. Since they are expensive, they are likely to be used for a number of years. Some of the films you may consider using will be outdated in one respect or another, but you can use them IF you alert the learners to disregard certain details.

8mm Film Loops

A film loop is a length of color movie film joined end to end and encased in a cartridge. This loop will run continuously until the projector is turned off. Silent film loops are short (up to five minutes) and rather inexpensive (about $20 per loop). Sound film loops are longer (usually 10 to 30 minutes) and more expensive (about $75 to $100 per loop).

Both silent and sound film loops may be used for both individual or group instruction; there is no threading of a projector—just insert the cartridge. Most film loops are commercially prepared, but film from a home movie camera may be edited and inserted into a film loop cartridge by a commercial movie lab.

The projector for a silent film loop is very small and light and is well suited for individual instruction. The projector for a sound film loop is quite large, but since no threading is required, it is useful in waiting rooms, clinics, and other group settings.

Books and Other Printed Materials

Depending upon the learner, printed material may be used in three ways: 1) in lieu of other forms of teaching, 2) to supplement other media, or 3) as an aid to review at a later time. The usefulness of printed materials depends upon the characteristics of the patient. It has been found, for example, that many white female college graduates are more likely to *read* information than to *listen* to it. Persons for whom English is a second language, on the other hand, are likely to have difficulty with teaching materials written in English.

You should consider three factors before using printed materials.

1. *Do not assume that your patient can read.* It is tragic, but true, that some high school graduates are unable to read above a third- or fourth-grade level and that there are many functional illiterates in this country. The nonreader is likely to be adept at concealing this deficiency, so careful detective work may be necessary. Watch for behavior such as the gracious acceptance of a brochure or pamphlet that is then set aside to be "read later," rapid or cursory attention to the material, an unusually long time spent "looking" at the material, the presence in the room of reading matter that is apparently never read (it may be there for appearance only), or vague responses to your questions about his reaction to the material. Granted, these behaviors may be noted in persons who are very literate, but the appearance of several in the same patient may alert you to the possibility that he can not read.

2. *Do not assume that your patient can see well enough to read.* An older person may be literate, but his eyesight may have failed so much that he is now unable to read. He may have left his glasses at home, his glasses may need to be changed, or he may need glasses, surgery for

cataracts, or treatment for glaucoma. The patient may tell you this, or he may exhibit behaviors similar to those of the patient who cannot read.

3. *Evaluate the reading level of the materials you are using.* A careful assessment of both your patient and the available printed material should enable you to match the learner to the appropriate educational matter. During the course of conversation, you could ask him what he likes to read. The fact that one patient reads the *National Enquirer* while another reads *The New York Times* and the *Christian Science Monitor* is more significant than the fact that both are high school graduates.

If you plan to use many printed materials, or if you plan to write your own materials, you would do well to purchase one of the guides to readability that can be found in almost any book store, so that you can be sure that the reading level of your material is appropriate for your patients, whether they are children, college graduates, or new literates.

In addition to readability, you need to evaluate printed materials in terms of style and format. If the style is dull, the type is small, and the page appears crowded with words, the patient is not likely to read the material.

USING AUDIOVISUAL AIDS

If AV aids are needed and warranted, you can enhance their effectiveness by following four guidelines.

1. *Preview Materials Before Using Them!*

A most distressing situation occurs when you find yourself in front of a group of people to whom you have just shown an unuseful, inappropriate, or unacceptable film. The catalogue description sounded as if the film would be perfect for the occasion, so you didn't preview it.

This situation occurs most frequently with 16mm films. Because of their cost, most 16mm films you use will be rented or borrowed and must therefore be ordered from catalogues. Other types of AV materials are likely to be more readily available and more easily previewed. Check the delivery time; if there is a possibility that you might receive a film only a short time before you are scheduled to use it, order it to arrive a day early so that you can preview it.

If it is absolutely impossible to preview a film or tape, be honest with your learners. Tell them *before* you use the materials, "I haven't seen (or heard) this material, so I can't guarantee that it will meet our needs."

Perhaps you will find a small segment of a film that is excellent. Limit your use to that segment. Better three minutes of valuable material than 25 minutes wasted. In terms of effective teaching, even though you paid for the whole thing, it is wasteful to show the other 22 minutes of inappropriate or nonuseful material.

2. Prepare for Trouble

Despite full and proper precautions, trouble often plagues the use of AV materials. I remember an AV convention in Atlantic City. Several hundred educators and AV specialists were assembled for a session that was based on an audiovisual presentation. There was only one problem—no one could make the projector work! Eventually another projector was brought in, but in the meantime we waited like any other audience. There were a few jovial cries—"Is there an AV man in the house?"—but the overall situation was similar to one that you yourself are likely to encounter one day.

When planning your class or presentation it would be well to prepare Plan A and Plan B (the disaster plan). Plan A is the way you expect to conduct the session; Plan B is what you will do if, at the last minute, you must proceed without your AV aids.

If the film fails to arrive, don't panic—go to Plan B. If you find when you preview the film that it will not help your presentation, do without. Go to Plan B. If the projector breaks down or the power goes off, go to Plan B. You will find yourself able to cope with such situations with equanimity and good humor if you have a contingency plan.

3. Prepare the Setting

There is no way to guarantee a trouble-free presentation, but the following suggestions will increase its probability.

Anticipate possible problems. The room may present problems, either structurally or because of faulty maintenance. Common difficulties include windows that cannot be darkened, a missing screen or one that will not pull down, and lack of a table or stand for the projector. Whenever possible, visit the room and check it over several days in advance. Locate the electrical outlets. It is hard to retain a calm composure while you search for an elusive outlet (the outlets in one room I teach in are under the radiators).

Arrive early so that you can familiarize yourself with the equipment. Focus it, adjust the sound. If you are not familiar with the equipment that will be available, don't hesitate to ask for an operator. When you order the projector, request an extra bulb for it, and, if you think you may need it, an extension cord.

If a problem arises, ask for help. Someone in the room is likely to volunteer, and while he or she tries to remedy the situation, you are free to proceed with the lesson or presentation. Otherwise, if you spend time fiddling with the equipment, it may be difficult to regain the group's attention.

4. Prepare the Learners

Tell them what to watch for. (What are the critical elements, the most important points? Is there some action or sound that might be missed? Tell them what it is and when it will occur.)

Tell them what to disregard. (Is the film outdated? Are there outdated fashions, slang phrases, and the like? Things that make a Hollywood period film authentic may not enhance a health film. There is a great difference between a *classic* Humphrey Bogart film and an *old* educational film.)

Identify possible differences from local practice or from what the audience have been taught if the difference might confuse their understanding of the rest of the film.

Indicate the nature of possible distractions, such as noticeable splices, a poor sound track, or noisy projector. The difficulty will not be remedied, but the audience will react differently if they know that you are aware of the problem but can do nothing about it.

Explain any aspect that might be frightening or anxiety-producing. In one childbirth film there is a shadow, possibly from the camera, across the baby as it is delivered. The baby does not cry immediately, and this, coupled with the shadow, makes one think the baby is dead. The viewers' response to the possibility of a dead baby is upsetting and an unnecessary detraction from an otherwise fine film.

5. Use the AV Material

Refer back to it during the remainder of your presentation. You expended considerable time, energy, and funds in order to use this AV material. Why did you do so? How can you justify its use? You did not incorporate AV material into your presentation merely to provide a pleasant interlude, so make sure that the learners understand and can use what they have seen and heard. You might select one or two incidents in the film as a basis for discussion: ask the audience whether they agree or disagree, and why. Or ask how the situation of a person in the film corresponds to what they have experienced to date. Regardless of your method, it is important to help your audience learn from the film and to integrate such learning into their response to your overall presentation and teaching.

EVALUATION OF AUDIOVISUAL MATERIALS

It is important that all AV materials be previewed before purchase or adoption for use. The catalogue description of educational materials cannot indicate the degree to which the producer's intentions coincide with your teaching needs, and often the description does not reflect the quality of the materials.

A form that includes the essential criteria for evaluation of educational materials is given in Appendix A. It is advisable for an agency or institution to keep a copy of each completed evaluation form for future reference. It is not uncommon for one or two persons to preview a set of materials but keep no record of the evaluation. A few months later another person may send for the same set of materials, not knowing that it has already been previewed and evaluated by persons within the same organization. Such duplication of effort decreases the effectiveness of patient education.

In addition to the criteria for evaluation in Appendix A, three points need special emphasis.

1. Check the producer's statement, if any, of intent, purpose, and objectives, as well as any suggestions for use. Decide how well the stated purposes, if any, coincide with your own teaching needs. The materials may be excellent for some teaching situations but not for yours.

2. Try to estimate how many patients, families, and other groups could benefit from the AV materials under consideration. It is difficult to meet the needs of many patients at once, when their learning needs and learning styles vary widely, but economy of use is often an important consideration. In what ways, if any, could the materials or their use be modified or supplemented to meet a variety of needs?

3. Remember that errors are possible in AV materials, even in those offered by the most reliable of producers and publishers! Never buy materials sight unseen unless you are prepared to correct and

compensate for possible errors with each and every group of learners.

If you do note errors or omissions as you preview instructional materials, it is helpful to send a detailed list of them to the publisher or producer; they may want to make corrections or include a list of errors with subsequent copies.

If you are involved in the purchase of AV materials, you will need to consider such factors as selection, operation, maintenance, and storage of both hardware and software. Appendix B lists some questions that you need to answer in selecting AV materials.

Before deciding on AV materials for a single purpose or group of learners, it would be well to think in terms of overall cost and use. For example, before deciding to invest in a slide-tape program to orient patients to the orthopedic unit of a hospital, the committee or persons involved might ask, "What are the orientation needs of other units?" "Could a slide-tape format be used for other programs, so that the equipment could have maximum use?" "Would any other format or medium, such as video tapes, be more useful throughout the hospital?"

Another approach would be to ask about the needs of related groups of patients and families. What teaching is needed by ALL preoperative patients regardless of diagnosis? What teaching needs do ALL patients on chemotherapy have in common? Which *general* teaching needs could be met with AV materials if the *specific* teaching needs were met through interaction with the nurse on the unit? Under what conditions would it be feasible to establish an AV library for patients and their families, using materials related to various conditions and diagnoses, as well as topics of general interest such as first aid, drug abuse, and hypertension? Just think what could be accomplished if the library cart in a hospital or extended care facility contained tape recorders and cassette tapes that patients could sign out for use by themselves and their families. Or if the waiting room of each clinic contained an everchanging selection of slides, tapes, and films for the use of patients and families.

In addition to planning for agencywide needs, it is desirable to consider community needs. In some communities, patient education might be achieved at a lower cost through an interagency exchange of materials that are important, expensive, and not needed frequently by any of the agencies involved.

Joint preparation of educational materials to meet local needs would extend the effectiveness of those persons most active in health education. For example, there is a limit to the number of presentations that can be given by a single nurse in a given year, but there is no limit to the number of persons who could learn from a taped or filmed presentation. As more and more homes acquire tape recorders, I can envision a section of each public library shelving cassette tapes, each offering an interesting lecture or discussion of a health problem or issue. These topics could range from biorhythms and nutrition to sex education and mental health and would benefit a wide variety of persons who might not attend the original presentation, such as self-conscious adolescents or homebound senior citizens.

There is no limit to the ways in which instructional technology can extend the effectiveness of your teaching. A significant improvement in health education in this country may come, not by adding more teachers, but by enabling enthusiastic, skillful teachers to reach more people.

YOUR PERSONAL AV FILE

Scarcely a week passes but I find something in a newspaper or magazine that helps me teach. The picture or article may describe a situation that will provoke discussion in class, give an example of a hard-to-teach concept, explain an abstract idea in simpler terms than I had thought possible, describe a new type of community self-help organization in another city, or include a picture or diagram to be saved for future use.

These items, saved over the years, are almost useless if dumped in a box or drawer, but are invaluable if filed for easy access. No matter how extensive your personal collection of educational materials may become, it will be of little use if you can't locate the materials easily or, worse yet, if you don't even know or remember what you have.

The following suggestions may help you develop a rich and useful file of educational materials.

1. *Decide upon a filing system.* As soon as you begin to collect materials, decide how you will catalogue them. You might categorize by disease, by nursing diagnosis, by categories used in various nursing indexes, or by a system of your own. The type of system used is less important than the fact that you have one. I find that I need to keep a key or index to my filing system because I haven't yet found a way to remember where I filed something that could easily be filed under

several categories. So, I keep a sort of Memory-Jogger list to help me find certain materials.

2. *Save, salvage, scrounge, clip, and collect.*   Keep a pair of scissors handy and cut out pictures and articles from magazines, newspapers, old textbooks, and advertising brochures. Save news of clubs, organizations, and agencies that your patients and families might contact for help. Xerox-copy materials that you cannot cut out. Save articles related to research on subjects of interest to you. Save pertinent book reviews and selected bibliographies, such as books that are useful in explaining death to children. Save single pictures; save printed matter ranging in length from a few sentences to a long article. Send for reprints such as the *Reader's Digest* series on the various organs and systems of Joe's body. Samples, models, and other three-dimensional objects can be catalogued and easily located by placing a "locator" slip in the appropriate manila folder, describing the item and telling where it is stored.

3. Sort and File Your Materials

For an investment of $10 you can buy approximately 100 manila folders, enough to last you for many years. As materials are placed in them, the labeled folders can be kept in a file drawer or a carton box, brightly painted or covered with wallpaper or contact paper.

As you file each item, it is important to date it and indicate its source. Such information is necessary when you periodically clean and sort your file, or if you want to seek more information on the subject.

4. Use the Materials

Refer to the materials for your own information, share them with patients, make Xerox copies to use in preparing booklets or pamphlets for your patients, and share the items with your colleagues as the occasion arises. As a safeguard against losing your materials, go to an office supply house or stationery store and buy a rubber stamp of your name, which will enable you to mark all your materials before you lend them to colleagues or patients. (I stamp the end and side of my books before I lend them—a visible marking on the outside is much more effective than a name on the inside.)

5. Sort, Select, and Discard at Intervals

Set aside an evening every month or so to file your most recent acquisitions. Since you have previously examined all these materials, the process of filing them can be done when you do not feel up to a more demanding task (some people can even file while watching television). In addition to saving materials, it is important to discard materials. By spending an afternoon each year discarding what is outdated or unwanted, you will keep your files in usable condition, a current asset in your professional activities.

16

Selected Aspects of Instruction

FEEDBACK

All of us seek information about ourselves, about the ways in which we affect other people, about the quality of our performance. We ask: "How did I do?" "What did you think?" "Was it OK?" "Did I do it right?" The information thus obtained enables us to monitor our behavior, maintaining or modifying it as needed.

In the terminology of systems theory, this information is called *feedback*; it is the portion of the output of a system that is fed back into the system. Feedback describes the performance of the system, enabling the system to maintain or correct itself.

The output of any component of the system may serve as feedback to that same component or to another one. In a teaching-learning situation, feedback may come from the learner, the teacher, or a product of the system, and may supply information to either the teacher or the learner or both.

Feedback to the Learner

Feedback may come to the learner, from the learner himself, in the form of subjective data. This information may be physiological, psychological, or both. It may indicate fatigue, anxiety, curiosity, disinterest, satisfaction, or any other reaction to learning. Given this feedback, the person learns how he is reacting to the situation.

Feedback may come to the learner in the form of objective data from some product or behavior that can be measured, from something he has done. The learner can compare this product or performance with a set of standards or criteria to determine what progress he has made. Examples of such products or performances would include the amount of weight lost, the score on a paper-and-pencil test, the accuracy of a return demonstration, or one's pulse rate after jogging.

Feedback may come to the learner from another person who has assessed the product or performance and who shares his observations and perceptions with the learner.

Feedback to the Teacher

Feedback to the learner is important; feedback to the teacher is equally important. The effectiveness of patient teaching depends largely upon the reaction of the learner, either positive or negative. This feedback enables you to decide whether to proceed, review, explain, or even drop the subject for the moment. An ongoing assessment of the learner's responses enables you to either maintain or modify your teaching approach. When you are teaching a child, his responses are often overt, and it is quite obvious when he does not understand you or when he has had enough for the time being. When you are teaching an adult, feedback related to your teaching may be more subtle, but it is equally as vital.

Positive and Negative Feedback

Feedback is neutral until it is compared with established criteria, norms, or a previous measurement. The data alone do not indicate a positive or negative state and cannot set a value of good or bad. For example, a test score of 132 is meaningless until it can be compared with the score that indicates a passing grade. A weight of 175 pounds means little until it is compared with the person's previous weight and with the norm for a person of similar build and height. If the comparison indicates a loss of 14 pounds, that feedback is neither positive or negative until you know whether the weight loss was intentional or whether it occurred despite the person's efforts to maintain his body weight.

Negative feedback indicates that the system has deviated from its normal functioning, and it is usually the basis for a change that will return the system to normal. Most biological regulation depends upon negative feedback, which redirects body functioning back toward the norm. Negative feedback opposes change and corrects deviations from the norm. Positive feedback, on the other hand, perpetuates deviations from the norm and is incompatible with biologic processes. For further information regarding feedback and body function, see the bibliography.

Feedback as Praise and Criticism

The terms positive and negative feedback are often used rather loosely with respect to teaching and learning. Positive feedback is usually synonymous with praise and negative feedback with criticism. When used in this sense, the terms seem to bear little relationship to systems theory. This use is not without foundation, however.

Criticism, when used effectively by a skillful teacher, helps to correct deviations from the norm and tends to redirect behavior back toward the established standards. Praise, like positive feedback, tends to reinforce movement away from the status quo and would tend to reinforce change. Although such continued movement away from homeostasis and equilibrium cannot be tolerated for bodily functions, it can result in continued movement and growth in the psychological and intellectual domains of activity.

With respect to learning, negative feedback consists of comments, responses, and reactions that would cause the learner to change his behavior to conform more closely to the established standards. Positive feedback in a learning situation includes those comments, responses, and reactions that reinforce the learner's behavior and that increase the likelihood that the behavior will be continued. Reinforcement will be described in detail in the next section.

Giving Feedback

Feedback is needed by and is often sought by the patient. The feedback you give the patient has the potential for being either helpful or harmful. The purpose of feedback is to supply information to the patient about his performance and about progress toward his objectives. Your praise or criticism must *describe the performance or progress* and must be carefully phrased to avoid any possibility of describing or labeling the patient himself. His wit, personal habits, charm, goodness, virtues, vices, mannerisms, and other attributes are irrelevant except as one or more of them may be affecting his learning. Even then, you will need to describe the effect of the attribute on the patient's learning and to avoid any labeling of his personality. Feedback that labels the person as good, smart, unresponsive, cooperative, slow, unmotivated, and the like is *not* helpful and is often harmful. Feedback that describes the patient's performance or behavior, rather than his personality, is helpful. Descriptions of performance or behavior give the patient the specific information he needs in order to improve, correct, or continue the behavior.

It is difficult to effectively phrase the feedback that you give your patients, but it is well worth the effort. The ability to give praise and criticism in a helpful, acceptable manner is useful not only in patient teaching; it is invaluable as you respond to your friends, family, and colleagues. See the bibliography for references that further explain the relationships among feedback, praise, and criticism.

REWARD AND REINFORCEMENT

"I tried it, but nothing happened—it's just not worth the effort." "I did my best—but it didn't make any difference, so why bother?" "Nobody seems to care, so why should I knock myself out trying?"

These statements reflect a universal desire for a satisfying outcome. No one can stand to be ignored or to feel that his actions have little effect or impact. We expect that whatever we do will have some effect, that it will make a difference. If the effect can't be a good one, a bad effect may be more satisfying than no effect at all. For example, to a child who feels ignored and unimportant, a scolding may be preferable to lack of attention. A scolding indicates that at least someone noticed what he was doing.

The absence of a satisfying outcome decreases a person's motivation or inclination to continue striving, eventually leading to a cessation of the effort. Conversely, a satisfying outcome rewards and reinforces the behavior, which in turn increases a person's motivation to continue. This cycle is true of patient teaching. Adequate reinforcement or reward increases the probability that the patient will keep on learning and that he will comply with prescribed therapy. Stated another way, the presence of a satisfying outcome reinforces the likelihood that the behavior will recur. The absence of a satisfying outcome lessens the probability that the behavior will recur. Therefore, the judicious use of reinforcement can markedly affect the probability that significant learning will take place.

Elementary school teachers have long used a system of rewards to foster learning. These rewards have ranged from gold stars to extra privileges. A reward for doing well is effective for persons who are able to do well, but a reward system is less effective with those who are not able to obtain the reward or win a prize. Therefore, reinforcement rather than reward is more useful in the teaching-learning process because it is applicable to all levels of performance and achievement.

To reinforce means to strengthen, and reinforcement refers to the process of strengthening a behavior, of increasing the probability that the behavior will recur. The process of reinforcement strengthens both desirable and undesirable behaviors. If a behavior elicits a response that is satisfying to the person who did it, he is likely to repeat it. This will happen whether or not the act is seen as desirable by other people. For example, antisocial acts may bring an adolescent the recognition by his peers that he was not able to obtain by socially acceptable means.

The Use of Reinforcement

The widespread effectiveness of reinforcement means that the person who is trying to reinforce the behavior of another person must be skilled and selective in using the process. All too often we focus on inept, incorrect or undesirable behaviors, and our attention tends to reinforce the very behaviors we would like to negate.

At the same time, our failure to acknowledge the expected, the correct, the desirable behavior can contribute to the extinction of those actions. This concept could be stated very simply as follows: Recognize the desirable, ignore the undesirable. This rule or guideline can be applied in many teaching situations, especially with respect to the affective domain. The community health nurse may use it as she teaches parents effective ways to interact with their children. For example, she can teach that consistent attention to a usually noisy child *when he is playing quietly* will promote quiet behavior more effectively than paying attention to him only when he is noisy. Consistent and caring attention paid to a demanding patient at times when his bell is *not* being rung is likely to prove effective in the long run in reducing the number of excessive demands.

Although reward and reinforcement of desired behavior is an effective teaching intervention, you cannot always afford to wait until the task is learned or accomplished. The patient is likely to become discouraged, to stop trying, to figure: "What's the use, I'll never make it." When the goal seems difficult or far away, encouragement and recognition of progress to date is crucial. Such encouragement and reinforcement is fairly common with motor behaviors such as crutch walking or learning to use a piece of equipment. It is less common in areas of social behavior, possibly because goals and objectives are not as clearly stated or as obvious.

If, for example, independence and active participation by the patient in the management of his illness are desired behaviors, then any move in that direction by the patient, no matter how small or seemingly insignificant, is worthy of reward and recognition. If all behaviors that contribute to that goal or objective are reinforced, the cumulative effect on the individual will be one of satisfaction, and he is likely to continue those behaviors. If it "feels good" to be a bit more involved in his own care, he is likely to become an increasingly active participant.

The nurse and family must be able to recognize any early, tentative movements toward the desired behavior in order to reward them. Therefore, the goals must be clearly and specifically stated. Otherwise, such movements might be misinterpreted. For example, the patient's tentative request to have physical therapy in the afternoon when he feels stronger rather than in the morning may be viewed as a complaint rather than as a desirable move toward active participation in planning his own care. If the request is viewed as a complaint, it may be refused and the patient may feel reprimanded. If the request is viewed as a desirable behavior, it can be reinforced. (The specific request need not be granted in order for the *act of requesting* to be supported and reinforced. The patient can be helped to feel that it was good to ask, even though, in this instance, the request could not be granted.)

Reinforcers. In the process of reinforcement, the object or condition that serves as a reinforcer will vary from person to person and situation to situation. Reinforcers can be verbal or nonverbal, material or intangible. They range from a cookie or M&M candy to a smile or hug, from extra privileges to increased responsibilities, from a verbal acknowledgment to a feeling of increased physical or mental well-being.

Some reinforcers are external and come from other people; others are internal and come from within. With respect to patient teaching, examples of inner reinforcement would include a sense of accomplishment, sleeping better, feeling good, increased self-esteem, an improved body image, and improved digestion. Some reinforcement can come both from within, and from other people who notice and comment upon such things as improved complexion, improved interpersonal relationships, a desired weight loss, or increased mobility.

The value of an agent or event as a reinforcer depends partly upon its meaning for the person and partly upon the satisfaction of basic needs. For a patient who has been NPO or on a limited diet, a less restricted diet may be a powerful reinforcer. The same diet could be seen as punishment to another patient who had previously enjoyed a completely free diet. For a patient whose lower-level needs have been met, reinforcers that help to meet his love and belonging or esteem needs are likely to be effective.

Guidelines for Reinforcing Desired Behavior

Since your contact with some patients or families may be brief, and opportunities for reinforcement may be limited, it is important that each opportunity be fully utilized. The following guidelines will help you provide reinforcement that is direct and effective.

Reinforcement must be overt and not merely implied.   The absence of a negative response may not be seen as a positive response or as intended reinforcement. The child whose mother has stopped scolding him may feel that she has stopped caring. The reinforcement or reward must be obvious, open, and *clearly identified* as a positive response.

Reinforcement must be specific for a given behavior.   If you nod and say "Great" at intervals throughout a community health visit, the family may sense approval on your part, but no specific behavior will have been reinforced. You will need to indicate whether you are approving and reinforcing progress toward a goal, a change in attitude, an accomplishment, or an initial attempt.

Reinforcement or reward must be justified.   Lavish praise, a phony enthusiasm, or unfounded approval have no place in the process of reinforcement. Only deliberate, genuine, positive acknowledgment of a desired behavior will be effective.

Vary the rewards.   Use different approaches and timing. An intermittent yet consistent pattern of reinforcement will be most effective. A single phrase or response, repeated ad nauseum with unvarying regularity, has virtually no power as a reinforcer. If, for example, increased ambulation is the desired behavior, a verbal acknowledgment, a nonverbal hug, or a shared "coffee break" are diverse responses that are likely to reinforce the patient's willingness to ambulate.

Reward promptly.   The effectiveness of reinforcement depends upon the promptness with which it is given. Even a short delay may render a reward ineffective with children or with a person whose memory or sense of time is impaired. The reward will be pleasant to receive, but its ability to influence behavior will have been drastically reduced by the delay.

Reward movement toward the desired behavior.   The process of reinforcing progress toward a desired behavior is specific and direct and is usually known to the patient. In some situations, however, it may be almost subliminal, with the patient being only vaguely aware of your deliberate and conscious reinforcement. This may occur with some children, persons who are confused or not fully conscious, and persons whose reasoning and ability to comprehend have been affected by illness, age, or medication. Despite differences in comprehension by the patient, this type of reinforcement rewards progress, sustains motivation, and encourages continued effort. In short, it helps the patient to "hang in there" and keep on trying.

Ignore undesired behavior whenever possible. Unless an undesired behavior is unsafe, disruptive, or illegal, it should be ignored whenever feasible. Behavior that is harmful or potentially harmful to the patient or others cannot be dismissed lightly, but other undesired behavior can be given as little attention as possible. It is important to remember that when the attention paid to undesirable behavior is greater than the reward or attention paid to desired behavior, the undesired behavior is reinforced. Complaining or demanding behavior, nonhelpful adaptations to pain (pain behaviors), noncompliance with prescribed regimens, and other negative responses can and should be overlooked IF adequate reinforcement is given for positive responses and desired behavior.

Supplement hidden rewards with verbal reinforcement. There is often a satisfactory, but not necessarily satisfying, outcome to continued compliance with prescribed therapy. A hypertensive patient who takes her medication regularly will be rewarded with a lowered blood pressure. She will be pleased by her doctor's comments during periodic checkups, but there may be little or no other reinforcement during years of conscientious compliance. The initial success is satisfying, but after a number of years without change, there may be little challenge and minimal motivation to continue. Invisible, physiological rewards that cannot be felt or experienced often need to be supplemented by your verbal recognition of a job well done.

REPETITION

In many situations, repetition is considered boring and undesirable. Even small children react to some kinds of repetition with remarks such as "You already said that" and "I heard you the first time." It is not surprising, then, that teachers often find it difficult to assume a positive attitude toward repetition and to deliberately repeat themselves as they teach.

Repetition is necessary for learning. In some situations the learner provides it for himself by rereading difficult material, recopying lecture notes, and repeating material that is to be memorized. In other situations the teacher must make provision for adequate repetition.

Repetition is needed if the material to be learned is completely new or difficult. Studies have shown that, on the average, two or three exposures to an idea are necessary before the material will seem familiar or be retained by the learner. Repetition in a lecture situation can be provided by an overview, presentation, and summary of the main ideas. Repetition of previously learned material, in the form of a review, may help in the learning of new material, especially if the old material was learned some time ago. Repetition, in the psychomotor domain, may take the form of practice. Repetition sometimes occurs as a simple reminder.

Repetition at a later date is needed when the patient or family is anxious or under great stress and is unable to hear and retain material as it is presented. Repetition at another time is needed when the patient or family is denying the present situation and is not ready to hear.

Despite the desirability of repetition within the teaching-learning process, you may at first tend to apologize for any repetition: "I don't like to repeat myself, but. . . ." "I know I already mentioned this, but. . . ." Since the effective use of repetition will be important to your patients, your challenge will be to provide repetition without being dull, boring, or apologetic.

Since you will be using repetition as a technique of teaching, it will be a conscious, deliberate action, one that you can learn to use effectively. First of all, assess the need for repetition through feedback from the patient or family. *You* may have presented the material only once, but several other people may have already given the patient the same information, and repetition has been provided. Or the idea may be so closely related to material previously presented that the patient was able to understand and retain it immediately. If the learner gives evidence of understanding, DON'T REPEAT.

Second, if repetition seems to be indicated, provide it, but creatively and skillfully. Repeat the main idea with a slight difference in words and in context. Use different phrases and different examples. The learner should recognize the idea, but view it in a different light. Many of the main ideas in this book have been repeated in different ways in several chapters. The repetition will have been successful if you found the material interesting and did not respond with a groan: "Oh, no! Not again!" Repetition is somewhat like salt. Nothing can quite replace it, but a little goes a long way.

PRACTICE

The amount of practice needed to develop a skill depends upon the capability of the learner, the complexity of the skill to be learned, and its similarity to existing skills of the learner. Learning to knit a given stitch may take hours of practice for a person who has never done any type of needlework. But it may take only a few minutes for an expert knitter who already has a repertoire of many, many knitting stitches.

If the skill to be learned is to replace a previously learned way of doing a task, considerable practice may be needed, because the person needs to unlearn one skill as he learns the one that is to replace it. This is especially true in the affective domain. A communication skill or interaction skill will require extensive practice if it is being learned as a replacement for an ineffective method of communicating or interacting. Since it often seems risky to change the ways in which we interact with other people, the initial practice of interpersonal skills should take place in a safe setting, such as a role-playing situation.

Practice and Feedback

Practice is useless without feedback and access to the criteria that describe a successful performance. The learner needs a basis for comparison, a standard to match. Feedback can come from the learner's comparison of his own performances. For example, he can tell that the piano scales sound better, or that his legs and wrists are less tired after crutch walking. Feedback may also come from someone else who observes the practice session (or the results of the practice) and gives a verbal evaluation. Practice without feedback may be nonproductive, because if the person does not know how well or how poorly he is doing, he is likely to perpetuate any mistakes he is making.

Practice and Reinforcement

The learner is unlikely to continue to practice without reinforcement. Whether the aim of practice is to play the piano or to walk with crutches, continuance depends upon a satisfactory outcome for the learner. For the child who is forced to practice the piano, a satisfactory outcome may be the absence of scolding, or completion of the practice in order to play. For the adult, a satisfactory outcome might be the ability to play increasingly complex tunes. In patient teaching, you may need to be ingenious in order to provide the reinforcement necessary to insure the amount of practice needed to develop a given skill.

Practice enables the patient to move closer to the desired level of competency. It is important that you and the patient be in accord regarding the level of performance that is desirable and the amount of practice that is needed; otherwise either you or the patient may be satisfied long before the other feels that the performance is acceptable.

PACING

Pacing refers to the structuring of a learning situation by the teacher so that the learner can proceed at his own pace or speed. Pacing is commonplace in academic settings, in which students are able to proceed through a curriculum at varying rates through the use of programmed instruction, independent study, self-instructional packets, and the like. Such opportunities are less common in patient teaching for two reasons: First, there is a lack of individualized educational materials. These materials are expensive and time-consuming to prepare. A single agency or institution usually cannot afford to develop such materials, and as yet there is no widely accepted "curriculum" for patient teaching that would facilitate commercial preparation of individualized instructional materials.

Perhaps an even greater obstacle to pacing is the sense of urgency that is often created by the nature of the patient's illness or condition and by the limited amounts of time available to the nurse for patient teaching. The nurse's teaching time seems especially brief when compared with the semester-long or year-long contact of teachers and learners in an academic setting.

Pacing and Patient Teaching

Although effective pacing may be difficult in patient teaching, it is important, and you will need to do the best you can to adjust your rate of teaching to the needs of each patient. The pace that is optimal for the patient depends upon the following factors.

Recency of previous study. A college student can probably learn more rapidly than a person who for many years has not consciously studied a topic or deliberately tried to learn a new skill.

Attention span. Is the patient psychologically and physically comfortable and able to concentrate for relatively long periods? Or is he uncomfortable and distractable?

Domains of learning. Some persons learn a motor skill more easily and more rapidly than they can learn abstract intellectual content. A person may learn very slowly in the affective domain if the skill or material to be learned seems risky or requires a major change in attitude.

Urgency, eagerness, and determination. If the reward or goal seems important and desirable, the patient may learn very rapidly.

Progress (or lack of progress). Pacing is affected by the patient's ability to tolerate frustration. You will know from your assessment of the learner whether he needs to learn in units that are small enough to insure success each step of the way, or whether he is able to cope with any discouragement and frustration that may occur.

Feedback, whether from a single patient or from a large audience, will help you to pace your teaching so that it is slow enough for effective and thorough learning, yet fast enough to maintain interest.

LANGUAGE

You may never have thought of yourself as a translator, but that is exactly the role you will need to assume in many situations before you can effectively teach the patient. There are two major groups of persons with whom there may be mutual problems with communication. The first group includes those who either do not understand English or for whom English is a second language. The needs of the person who does not speak English are rather dramatic and urgent, and an interpreter is usually found without delay. The problems of persons for whom English is a second language may be far more serious with respect to patient teaching, simply because they may not be recognized and therefore are not dealt with. These patients and their families may need help in understanding the doctor and nurse and in finding words to describe their symptoms or explaining changes in body function. They may need help in learning how to interact with doctors and nurses, in learning how to assume the "sick role" in an unfamiliar culture. You can help a person for whom English is a second language by making your willingness to help overt and specific. Ask what behaviors on your part would be helpful. Does the person want you to be patient and wait when he seems to be struggling to find a word, or would it be more helpful for you to supply the word he may not know? The important thing is that you recognize the problem and verbalize your willingness to help, rather than ignoring the problem or assuming that it does not exist.

The second group of persons with whom you may have difficulty communicating are those native-born Americans who understand and speak English, but who speak in a language that sounds foreign to you. Such groups include patients and families who use the language of the streets, earthy gutter language with which you may be unfamiliar. Some adolescents and young adults seem to be speaking a foreign language even though each individual word is familiar. Senior citizens may use words and phrases of a different era, the precise meanings of which are not clear to you.

This problem cannot be lightly dismissed, because, in order to teach, you must be able to communicate. The energy you must expend to help these patients understand you may be equal to or greater than your effort in communicating with persons who do not understand English at all. You will need to be overt in your desire to understand, and ask for clarification whenever you do not fully understand. As you work to learn the language of various groups of patients, it may be helpful to compile a list of synonyms for various body parts and functions; this may be useful in future teaching.

Guidelines for Facilitating Communication

Besides conscientiously using your basic communication skills, there are several ways you can increase the effectiveness of your interaction with groups for whom language may be a problem.

Assume responsibility for sending a clear message.   The sender of a message is responsible for its clarity. If an unclear message is not understood, it is not the fault of the receiver. For example, if a naval officer gives a graduation address to his home-town high school in semaphore, it is not the fault of the students that they cannot understand it. A professor of sociology who is opening a new senior citizen housing project might base his remarks on systems theory, using such terms as entropy, negentropy, and equifinality, in order to stress the interrelatedness of all segments of society. The majority of the senior citizens present may not understand him, but the failure to communicate lies with the professor, not with the senior citizens.

Your message will be clearer and your teaching more understandable if you use good basic English and consistently eliminate all professional jargon and abbreviations.

Watch for clues that indicate the message is not clear. Look for nonverbal cues that indicate that the patient does not understand your message—a frown, a puzzled look, a failure to respond, or letting the subject drop. Listen for verbal cues that the patient was not able to understand your message—an inappropriate response or a remark that doesn't quite fit.

Communicate any lack of understanding on your part without blaming the patient. The patient may not be sending a clear message because of discomfort, fatigue, confusion, anxiety, or any of many other stressors. You can help by asking him to clarify so that you can better understand him. Gentle, nonthreatening questions convey the fact that you don't understand without making the patient feel awkward or foolish: "I'm not sure I understand." "Do you mean . . .?" "Is that the same as . . .?" Responses that blame the patient tend to inhibit any meaningful communication: "Say what you mean." "You are not making sense." "You are not expressing yourself clearly at all." In contrast, the simple phrase, "I don't think I understand," can facilitate further conversation.

Rephrase your message as often as necessary for understanding. You may need to search for synonyms and alternate phrases as you provide the repetition that the patient needs for complete comprehension. Rephrase your message as often as necessary to get a confirmation of understanding from the patient that: a) you understand him, and b) he understands you. This confirmation may be verbal or nonverbal. Examples of verbal confirmation include: "Yes, that's what I mean," "Oh, I see," and "Oh, now I understand."

Do's and Don't's

Do use language with *skill*, based on a careful assessment of the patient. Communicate with each patient as an individual and avoid the sloppy pattern of dropping down to the level of the least common denominator of communication. Retain (or develop) the ability to use language appropriately so that you can communicate with an engineer as effectively as with a child, with a senior citizen as effectively as with a juvenile delinquent.

Street language may be necessary, appropriate, and useful in some situations, while in others it may be inappropriate and may in fact alienate you from the very persons you are trying to teach.

Never talk down—don't be condescending. Never talk up—don't be pretentious.

Don't tease or make jokes unless the lines of communication are open and effective. Well-intentioned teasing and joking is often the basis for hurt and misunderstanding. How many times have you heard a person try to rectify an error by saying, "But I was only teasing!" or "Couldn't you tell that I was only joking?" Your time with your patient is too important to waste on unproductive interactions or potentially harmful ones such as teasing.

Don't be phony or artificial in your use of language. You do not need to talk babytalk to communicate with a child. You do not need to swear to communicate with a seemingly tough runaway adolescent. Your use of language should be appropriate to the situation and should represent a sincere desire to communicate with the person whom you are trying to teach.

THE TEACHING-LEARNING PROCESS

EVALUATION

17

Evaluation

Evaluation is an inevitable, unavoidable, integral part of life. All day long, day in and day out, each of us is involved in it. Evaluations are made, one after another, as we answer questions such as: Is this product living up to the advertiser's claim? Is my congressman doing a good job? Are the beans ripe enough to pick? Is the baby developing normally? And so on.

Evaluation is easy if the standards or criteria are objective and precise. If it takes a yard of material to make an apron, it is not difficult to determine whether a piece of fabric is big enough for an apron; we simply measure it with a tape or yardstick.

Evaluation is not easy if the criteria are vague or completely subjective. Is the dress pretty? The answer depends on so many things that it is almost impossible to give an unqualified yes or no answer.

Evaluation is often hard when people are involved, especially when an abstract concept such as learning is to be evaluated. A patient's height, weight, and body temperature can be accurately measured and precisely evaluated, but not a person's communication skills or manual dexterity.

EVALUATION AND PATIENT TEACHING

Two aspects of teaching should be evaluated regularly: teaching effectiveness and teacher performance. They are closely related, but we can evaluate them separately.

Teaching effectiveness is based upon the objectives established and is evaluated in terms of patient learning. Teacher performance is based upon both the teacher's personal objectives and external standards for instructional skills.

The pages that follow describe the evaluation of teaching effectiveness and teacher performance, giving general considerations plus specific methods of evaluation for each.

EVALUATION OF TEACHING EFFECTIVENESS

Teaching effectiveness depends on patient learning and is evaluated through periodic assessments of the patient's progress and accomplishments. This process describes what the patient has learned and identifies what he still needs to learn. It tells you and the patient how far he has come and how far he has to go in order to meet the objectives that have been set. It is not an easy process, because in many situations the objectives are not clear. Unless you and the patient have a clear idea of what must be learned, neither of you will be able to be sure that it has in fact been learned.

Objectives serve as a road map for the process of evaluation. They enable you and the patient to identify your goal or destination, to trace your progress toward that goal, and to tell when you have arrived. Together you will be able to evaluate the learning that has taken place and to obtain a clear idea of what remains to be learned.

Evaluation and Instruction

The process of teaching includes both evaluation and instruction. They are both integral parts of patient teaching, but they are different activities. Evaluation is the assessment of learning that has taken place. Instruction is the process of helping the patient to learn. Although they are interrelated, instruction and evaluation are distinct processes and should be kept separate. The patient should know which one is taking place at any given time.

During a period of instruction, the patient is free to learn, to question, to make mistakes, to practice, to expose his lack of knowledge or understanding. He is not expected to KNOW; he is in the process of LEARNING. During a period of evaluation, however, learning is momentarily suspended as the patient demonstrates in some way how much he has learned, and how well he understands the material. The results of this evaluation serve as feedback to both you and the patient and give direction to future learning and teaching.

The frequency with which evaluation takes place depends upon the nature and amount of material to be learned, the amount of time available, and the way in which the patient learns best. Your previous assessments of the patient will have indicated whether evaluation should be part of each teaching session or whether it should take place at a separate time. If the material to be learned is difficult and complex, you may choose to pause every five to 10 minutes to evaluate the patient's understanding. Or you may decide, for example, to spend the last 10 minutes of a visit to the patient's home in evaluating the family's understanding and ability to care for him.

Evaluation and the Patient

Regardless of which approach you take, the patient needs to know how and when you plan to evaluate. In most situations you will not use the word evaluation but will say something like: "Let's talk about your diet for awhile, and then I'll ask you some questions to find out if I have explained it clearly." Or, "Here is a list of your medications, and the doses and effects. First, I'll explain them, and then you study them. I'll be back tomorrow and will ask you to tell me what they are without looking at the paper." Or, "I'll demonstrate the procedure for you and tell you what I'm doing. Then I'll do it again and stop every few minutes so you can tell me how well you understand the reasons for each step."

The most important concept in evaluation, in my opinion, is that the person is more important than the performance or the product. Regardless of how well he has done, it is imperative that you help the patient maintain his dignity and his self-esteem throughout the process of evaluation. He may have learned very little, but he is not a failure. He may give a failing performance, but he is not a failure. The behavior may fail to reach the objective, but the person is not a failure.

It is inexcusable, in my opinion, to evaluate any person in such a manner that he feels dumb, stupid, inept, put down, or inferior. I feel that the psychological damage done to a patient by lessening his self-confidence and self-esteem is equal to, or greater than, any physical damage that can be inflicted by negligence or mistreatment. Within the health care delivery system the potential for psychological harm is great, because first, the patient often views the nurse as an authority figure, and second, a person is more vulnerable when he is ill. I would go so far as to suggest that anytime a patient is hurt during the evaluation process, whether by accident or intent, the nurse is guilty of a form of malpractice.

People grow on the basis of successes, not failure, and your evaluation can be structured to indicate areas of successful learning. If the patient feels good about what has been accomplished to date, he is likely to resume learning with renewed vigor. He will want to know how much remains to be accomplished, and how he can proceed to reach his goal. Once he knows this, you can make realistic plans together.

Evaluation of Learning

Some of the methods of evaluation that are useful in an academic setting are not feasible for patient teaching, but fortunately other means are available. A few of the most commonly used methods include written tests, oral evaluation, return demonstrations, physical findings, and questionnaires.

Written tests.   Paper- and-pencil tests have a limited usefulness in patient teaching, because it is difficult and time-consuming to construct a test that is valid and reliable for use with a wide range of patient capabilities. Most tests are prepared for a specific group of learners and for a specific grade or college level. It is not practical to construct a separate test for each patient, and it would be extremely difficult to prepare a test related to cancer, for example, that would be valid for many patients with a wide variety of educational backgrounds, experiences with cancer, and learning objectives. Difficulty in preparation does not preclude the use of tests in patient teaching, however.

If you plan to become involved in test construction, you will need to learn how. Get a good book on test construction, take a course, or enlist the aid of an expert. Before you actually use your test in patient teaching, administer it to a variety of people in order to discover and correct problems related to directions, clarity of questions, ease of scoring, and so on. Compare the test scores with some other indicator of learning for a rough measure of reliability. If you feel certain that the patient has learned a great deal and has met a set of objectives but he receives a very low test score, something is wrong.

Tests may be more useful with groups of learners than with an individual patient. A pretest, given several weeks before your lecture to a group that meets regularly, can give you valuable information about the group's current level of understanding and provide a basis for planning your lecture.

A pretest is given for one of two reasons. First, it may be given to obtain data for assessing the learner and formulating objectives. A pretest helps to determine "where the learner *is at.*" If a test is given for this purpose, be sure to *use* the information. It is a waste of time and energy to administer a test that is just filed away.

Second, a pretest is used with a posttest to evaluate learning. The difference between the two scores or responses indicates the learning that took place between the taking of the two tests.

A single test, given at the end of a period of learning, provides feedback to both learner and teacher. Minimal emphasis should be placed on the test score, however. A high score may mean that the patient has truly learned all the essential material, but it may also indicate that the test was very easy or that the patient is a skilled test taker. A low score may indicate minimal learning, or it may indicate either a poorly constructed test or an anxious patient who is a poor test taker. If valid and reliable tests are available, they may be used by the patient for self-evaluation.

Oral evaluation. A portion of each teaching session, or a special period of time, can be set aside for an oral evaluation of the patient's learning. Instead of giving the patient a written test, you can ask him questions that, if answered correctly, will indicate learning. For many patients, such an evaluation will need to be structured more like a discussion than an examination. If the patient has not been tested or examined since his school days, a more formal evaluation may be very threatening.

Your evaluation of some patients must be especially gentle, seemingly casual, and supportive. The expected changes in behavior may be more difficult or threatening to the patient than you could ever imagine, and your responsibility as a teacher must be to support the patient through what may be a major crisis for him as he tries to learn a new way of relating to himself and his world.

When assessing learning, whether by written test or oral questioning, a combination of broad and narrow questions will be useful. A narrow question with a right or wrong answer, such as "What is the name and dose of each medication you will take when you go home?," will indicate how much the patient can remember of what he has been taught. Broad questions, such as "What would you do if . . .?" or "What do you think would happen if . . .?," will help you assess the patient's ability to use the material he has learned and to solve problems related to his condition.

Return demonstration. The patient's ability to perform a given task or to demonstrate a skill without assistance will indicate learning. However, in any task or procedure, a perfect performance by the patient is less important than his ability to recognize and correct a mistake, should one occur. Accidents, errors, and mistakes are bound to happen sooner or later, and the patient's ability to compensate is much more significant in most situations than his ability to show you a single perfect performance. If the return demonstration was error-free, it would be good to follow it up with a discussion based on questions such as, "What would you do if you dropped the . . .?" or "What would you do if you couldn't reach the . . .?"

Analysis of physical findings.   In some situations you can evaluate learning on the basis of objective data from your own observations or laboratory tests. You may conclude that the patient has learned and that the objectives have been met if you can document such things as planned weight loss, normal blood sugar, decreased or normal blood pressure, increased tolerance of ambulation, or absence of complications.

Subjective findings, reported by the patient, such as increased vigor, improved appetite, and greater well-being may also indicate that significant learning has taken place.

Follow-up questionnaire.   You can obtain useful information about learning and the long-range effectiveness of your teaching by the use of a well-constructed questionnaire. I specify well-constructed because the development of an effective questionnaire requires considerable skill. It is exciting to analyze the information obtained from a clear, precise, complete questionnaire; it is frustrating and disappointing to realize that one's questionnaire is yielding little useful information. Consult the library, the faculty of a nearby college or university, or the research department of your agency for assistance in developing a productive questionnaire.

A questionnaire is often sent to patients a month or two after the end of the patient teaching sessions, and a second one may follow in six to 12 months. The information sought is usually related to hoped-for, or desired, behavioral changes rather than specific knowledge or information. The questions are shaped to reveal changes in life style or attitude, compliance with therapeutic regimens, adherence to protocol or established procedure, and areas of concern or difficulty. The data from a follow-up questionnaire are used to modify current teaching programs for the benefit of future patients, or to plan follow-up sessions for the original group of patients.

EVALUATION OF TEACHER PERFORMANCE

The feedback you receive about your teaching will enable you to increase your competency as a teacher. You will need to take the initiative to get this information—you will need to seek it deliberately and systematically, but once you have begun to do so, your patients and colleagues are often willing to help you improve your teaching skills.

During your first few years of teaching or your initial experiences with a new method of teaching, it is helpful to prepare two sets of objectives. One set, the objectives for the patient's or audience's learning, are related to *what* you are trying to teach. The second set, your personal goals for a given teaching experience, are related to *how* you are trying to teach. The first set of objectives forms the basis for an evaluation of learning and teaching effectiveness; the second set forms the basis for an evaluation of your teaching performance.

An example of an objective for patient learning might be: Each patient will be able to explain the benefits of coughing and turning postoperatively.

If, in the past, you have tended to forget to provide an opportunity for practice, your personal teaching objective might be: I will remember to have each patient practice coughing enough times to be sure that he will be able to do it with minimal discomfort after surgery.

Given these objectives, when you ask your patient to evaluate your teaching, you will be able to ask, very specifically, "Did I help you to practice coughing enough before surgery to enable you to do it after surgery with minimal discomfort?" The answer to such a specific question will be useful, but the answer to a vague question such as "Was I helpful to you before surgery?" is not likely to be useful at all.

If you are to give a talk to a community group, your personal objective might be to decrease the number of times you say "OK?" or "UH. . . ." Another personal objective might be to repeat each question from the audience before answering it so that the audience can benefit from the answer. You may or may not want to ask the audience for an evaluation, but you can tape your speech and evaluate it in terms of your personal objectives in the privacy of your home.

Ways to Evaluate Your Teaching Performance

As much as you may need and want an evaluation of your performance as a teacher, it is not easy to seek it nor is it easy for others to give. In describing ways to evaluate your teaching performance, I will start with the ones that are likely to seem the least risky, and therefore the easiest and safest to use.

Feedback from a recording of the situation. An audio tape will enable you to listen to yourself in the privacy of your own home or office. The tape recording can be made inconspicuously, although if you are recording a group discussion, you may need to ask permission of the group or tell them the reason and purpose for recording the session.

First, listen and react to the tape as a whole. You will probably hear things you didn't even know you said. Then, listen to the tape with reference to your personal objectives. Compare what you intended to do, or what you were trying to do, with what you actually said and did. You may be dismayed, surprised, or pleased, but whatever your reaction, you will have a basis for either maintaining or modifying your teaching for your next presentation.

If you have access to a videotape recorder, use it as soon as possible. You and your patients will be very much aware of it at first, and you may feel self-conscious, but by the end of that teaching session, or after a few more sessions, you will be able to ignore it. The video tape will enable you to examine your nonverbal behavior—such things as your posture, the frequency with which you smile (or frown), your tendency to move about or stand still, and the presence of any distracting mannerisms.

Written feedback from learner.   A printed or dittoed evaluation form is useful in obtaining feedback from either a large group or a single patient. It is usually anonymous and can be returned to you at the end of a class, left at the desk by a patient upon discharge, or mailed back to you at a later date.

The evaluation form may include open-ended questions, a checklist or rating scale, or multiple-choice questions. The form of each question is less important than its specificity. The usefulness of the information you receive depends upon your ability to ask for what you need and want. You will need to be specific, clear, and direct, because a vague question usually elicits a vague answer. In general, an answer can be no better than the question.

Here are two examples of specific open-ended questions: "What did I do that was helpful to you in learning to . . .?" "What could I have done to help you learn more easily (or quickly)?"

Ask the patient for specific information related to your performance as a teacher. Ask about the things that are of concern to you, such as interest, pacing, organization, use of humor, poise, and tone of voice.

When your evaluation forms are returned to you, take each one seriously, but do not overreact to any single evaluation! A "bad" or "poor" evaluation is disturbing, but while it may be realistic and accurate, there is always the possibility that the writer was upset or angry with something other than your teaching. The overall pattern of responses will give you a more accurate description of your teaching than will an isolated evaluation or two, whether favorable or unfavorable.

Direct feedback from patient or colleagues. Often your most helpful feedback will come directly from a patient or colleague, perhaps during an informal conference or a conversation over a cup of coffee. But the process of getting such feedback can be difficult. If you feel that your teaching performance was acceptable or good, you may feel as if you are fishing for compliments when you ask someone to evaluate it. If your teaching performance was poor or unsatisfactory, your patient or colleague may feel put on the spot when you ask him about it. The evaluation process is affected by the nature of your relationship with the person who will evaluate you. For many people, the closer the relationship, the harder it is to give and receive feedback.

The evaluation process can be made somewhat easier for all concerned if you share your objectives, in writing, with the other person. Your written personal objectives will facilitate direct evaluation in three ways. First, they structure the conference or conversation. Objectives provide a specific starting point, and they tend to keep the interaction focused upon what you were trying to do and what you actually did. Second, objectives tend to elicit useful information. You obtain feedback about the things that are of concern to you rather than about extraneous aspects that are easy to talk about. Third, objectives tend to protect you from unnecessary and unhelpful comments about your personality. Objectives help your evaluator to describe your performance and not your personality.

If you want to profit from evaluation data and use them for professional growth, it is important to be specific when discussing your teaching performance. It is not very helpful to know only that a given behavior was "good." You will need to ask your patient or colleague, "What made it good?" "How do you know it was good?" "How could you tell?" You need to know the answers to such questions so that, deliberately and intentionally, you can repeat at a later date the behavior that was good. Unless you can identify and describe these successful behaviors, your teaching performance can improve only by chance or circumstance, because you won't know what you did or how you did it.

The most important ingredient of direct feedback from a patient or colleague is mutual respect and trust. There must be an openness and willingness to share, with no suspicion of retaliation at a later date. If you seek an evaluation from a person with whom you have not yet developed a trusting relationship, it is important that this person not be dependent upon you. For example, it is not fair to ask a patient who is dependent upon your care for an evaluation of your teaching, if he feels that his comments might displease you and jeopardize his care. Such an evaluation would need to be done close to the end of your relationship.

In conclusion, evaluation is an integral part of the teaching-learning process, and it should be done frequently by the beginning teacher and at periodic intervals by the experienced teacher. Although evaluation of your teaching can be difficult, it can also be stimulating and satisfying, since it has the potential for facilitating professional growth and promoting self-actualization.

Bibliography

Chapter 1: TEACHING AND LEARNING

1. Fuerst, Elinor V.: The Nurse as a Health Teacher, Chap. 16 in *Fundamentals of Nursing.* 5th. ed.; Philadelphia, J. B. Lippincott Company, 1974, pp. 147–56.

   Presents principles of learning and implications for teaching. Briefly presents concepts related to objectives, content, evaluation, environment, and methods of teaching.

2. Redman, Barbara Klug: *The Process of Patient Teaching in Nursing.* 3rd ed.; Saint Louis, The C. V. Mosby Company, 1976, 272 pages.

   Comprehensive treatment of patient teaching, including a chapter on the delivery of patient education. Extensive references.

3. Rogers, Carl R.: *Freedom to Learn.* Columbus, Charles E. Merrill Publishing Company, 1969, 358 pages.

   Parts I and II present practical ways to stimulate and facilitate *significant* learning. Part III gives the conceptual framework and Part IV presents the personal and philosophical aspects of the concept of "freedom to learn."

4. Schweer, Jean E.: Teaching Students to Teach Health Care to Others. *Nurs. Clin. North Am.* 6(4):679–90 (Dec. 71).

   Pages 681–90 present concepts relevant to patient teaching, including 12 conditions that facilitate learning, as well as ways to vitalize demonstrations, overcome language barriers, and use television.

5. Sturdevant, Bonnie: Why Don't Adult Patients Learn. *Superv. Nurse* 8:44, 46 (May 77).

   Brief overview of teaching-learning process including assessment of learner, selection of content and method, motivation, role of family, and evaluation.

Chapter 2: AN OVERVIEW OF PATIENT TEACHING

6. Bivin, Victoria E.: The Clinical Specialist—An Educator. Some Problems and a Possible Approach. *Nurs. Clin. North Am.* 8(4):715–21 (Dec. 73).

   Describes role of clinical specialist in both staff and patient education. Stresses importance of good setting for both groups in response to need of adult learners.

7. Green, Lawrence W.: The Potential of Health Education Includes Cost Effectiveness. *Nurs. Digest* 8:64–7 (Spring 78).

   Describes nine general goals or benefits of health education. The author believes that benefits far outweigh the costs.

8. Grout, R. E., and Watkins, J. D.: The Nurse and Health Education. *Int. Nurs. Rev.* 18(3):248–57 (1971).

   Reviews changes made and needed in health education, and factors involved in planning learning experiences. Discusses process of working with individuals, groups, and communities toward behavior change. Discusses process of evaluation. Gives examples.

9. Henry, Agnes P.: The Role of Women's Magazines in Health Education. *Nurs. Times* 65:1280–1, 2 (Oct. 69).

   Nurse journalist describes process of producing an article on health in a magazine. Describes role of women's magazines (two magazines received a total of 76,000 letters in one year asking for information on health matters).

10. Levin, Lowell S.: Patient Education and Self-Care: How Do They Differ? *Nurs. Outlook* 26:170–5 (March 78).

    Draws sharp distinctions between patient education and self-care education. Describes ways in which they are antagonistic and indicates ways in which they could be complementary. Very thought-provoking.

11. Murray, R., and Zentner, J.: Guidelines For More Effective Health Teaching. *Nursing '76* 6:44–53 (Feb. 76).

    Lively presentation of practical suggestions for teaching, conditions for learning, the role of language, culture, and age, techniques of teaching, prohibitors in the teaching-learning process, follow-up teaching, and health promotion.

12. Palm, Mary Lock: Recognizing Opportunities for Informal Patient Teaching. *Nurs. Clin. North Am.* 6(4):669–78 (Dec. 71).

    Pages 671–5 describe a study of the priority of patient teaching. Pages 675–8 describe identification of informal teaching opportunities, and teaching during nursing care.

13. Powell, A. H., and Winslow, E. H.: The Cardiac Clinical Nurse Specialist—Teaching Ideas that Work. *Nurs. Clin. North Am.* 8(4):723–32 (Dec. 73).

    Brief philosophy of teaching and learning followed by discussion of teaching patients and of inservice education for nurses on ways to teach patients; theoretical concepts plus useful examples.

14. Redman, Barbara K.: Guidelines for Quality of Care in Patient Education. *Can. Nurse* 71(2):19–21 (Feb. 75).

    Author states that "the age of patient education is upon us, and we're not ready." Suggests process for documenting need for teaching and developing a priority system for meeting patient education needs.

15. Redman, Barbara K.: Patient Education as a Function of Nursing Practice. *Nurs. Clin. North Am.* 6(4):573–80 (Dec. 71).

    Describes current status of patient teaching by nurses, discusses teaching skills and developments needed in patient education.

16. Schweer, S., and Dayani, E.: The Extended Role of Professional Nursing—Patient Education. *Int. Nurs. Rev.* 20(6):174–5 (1973).

    Examines existing problems in the patient education provided by nurses, and offers suggestions for clarifying nurse's role and improving patient education.

17. Skeen, Carole: We made Teen-Age Health Care Free—But It Wasn't Easy. *RN* 39:38–40 (July 76).

    Describes the development of a free clinic in Detroit staffed by professional and nonprofessional volunteers to provide medical care and counseling for adolescents and young adults.

18. Smith, Carol R.: Patient Education in Ambulatory Care. *Nurs. Clin. North Am.* 12(4):595–607 (Dec. 77).

    Identifies and describes eight reasons for lack of patient teaching. Describes the process of initiating, developing, and implementing a structured teaching program, including administrative aspects.

19. Winslow, Elizabeth H.: The Role of the Nurse in Patient Education. Focus: The Cardiac Patient. *Nurs. Clin. North Am.* 11(2):213–22 (June 76).

    Cites research that presents positions about patient teaching held by patients, nurses, and physicans. Lists eight factors identified by nurses as interfering with patient teaching.

Chapter 3: SYSTEMS THEORY AND NURSING

20. Craven, R. F., and Sharp, B. H.: The Effects of Illness on Family Functions. *Nurs. Forum* 11(2):186–93 (1972).

Describes the impact of illness upon the structure, functions, and roles within the family. Briefly describes ways in which nursing can help to support family functions.

21. Hazzard, Mary E.: An Overview of Systems Theory. *Nurs. Clin. North Am.* 6(3):385–93 (Sept. 71).

    Defines and describes systems in general. Discusses concepts in system theory, including matter and energy, information, self-regulation of systems, and feedback. Briefly discusses the use of models. Basic theory with little application. References.

22. Hazzard, M. E., and Scheuerman, M.: Family System Therapy: New Way to Help Families in Trouble. *Nursing '76* 6:22–3 (July 76).

    Case study shows how systems theory can give insight into behavior of a family and provide a basis for therapy.

23. Moughton, Mona, and Hazzard, Mary: Systems Theory and the Adolescent, in Duffy, M., et al., eds., *Current Concepts in Clinical Nursing,* Vol. 3. St. Louis, The C. V. Mosby Company, 1971, pp. 14–25.

    Detailed application of systems theory to the developmental process of adolescence. Helpful in increasing one's understanding of both systems theory and adolescence. Extensive references and bibliography.

24. Moughton, Mona, and Hazzard, Mary: Systems Theory and the Aged, Chap. 4 in Duffy, M., et al., eds., *Current Concepts in Clinical Nursing,* Vol. 3. St. Louis, The C. V. Mosby Company, 1971, pp. 26–36.

    Explores relationship between entropy and aging, and explains the processes and problems of elderly persons in terms of systems theory. Extensive references and bibliography.

25. Petrillo, Madeline, and Sanger, Sirgay: 8 Types of Families . . . and How They Affect Your Job. *Nursing '73* 3:43–7 (May 73).

    Describes ways in which interactions within the family system affect the nurse's relationship with the hospitalized child.

26. Shepard, K., and Barsotti, L.: Family Focus—Transitional Health Care. *Nurs. Outlook* 23(8):574–7 (Sept. 75).

    Patient and family spend last few days of patient's hospitalization in a cottage learning skills that will be needed at home. Discharge plans based on use of the family support system.

Chapter 4: MASLOW AND PATIENT TEACHING

27. Goble, Frank G.: The Third Force—the Psychology of Abraham Maslow. New York, Pocket Books, 1970, 208 pages.
Presents a condensation of Maslow's ideas in a systematized and simplified organization, with the preface written by Maslow himself. Readable, interesting, useful introduction to Maslow's own writings.

28. Hanlon, Kathryn: Maintaining Sexuality after Spinal Cord Injury. Nursing '75 5:58–62 (May 75).
Encourages nurses to include sexuality in early treatment as well as in rehabilitation. Acknowledges difficulties that both patient and nurse may experience in helping patient to meet this basic need.

29. Hatton, Jean: Performance Evaluation in Relation to Psychosocial Needs. Supervisor Nurse 8:30, 32, 35 (July 77).
Written with respect to staff evaluation, but the listing of specific helpful and nonhelpful behaviors gives nurse direction in trying to meet psychosocial needs of patients.

30. Johnson, Dorothy E.: Powerlessness: A Significant Determinant in Patient Behavior? J. Nurs. Educ. 6:39–44 (Apr. 67).
Uses research findings to support possible relationship between powerlessness and learning, especially in area of motivation.

31. Katona, Elizabeth A.: Learning Colostomy Control. Amer. J. Nurs. 67(3):534–41 (Mar. 67).
Illustrates interrelatedness of physical and psychological aspects of colostomy control. Does not refer specifically to Maslow's hierarchy of needs, but integrates the concepts throughout.

32. Luckmann, J., and Sorenson, K.: What Patients' Actions Tell You about Their Feelings, Fears and Needs. Nursing '75 5:54–61 (Feb. 75).
Describes factors that influence reactions to illness and 12 specific reactions to illness. Last three pages describe basic needs from survival through self-actualization.

33. Luckmann, J., and Sorenson, K. C.: Worries Illness Brings, Chap. 11 in Medical-Surgical Nursing—A Psychophysiologic Approach. Philadelphia, W. B. Saunders Company, 1974, pp. 70–3.
Illness interferes with the satisfaction of basic needs and creates worry and concern. Discusses ways in which illness can affect each level of needs in Maslow's hierarchy.

34. Maslow, Abraham H., Motivation and Personality. 2nd ed.; New York, Harper & Row, 1970, 369 pages.

Chapters 3–5 (pp. 19–75) introduce and expand upon Maslow's hierarchy of needs and his theory of human motivation.

35. Meyer, Herbert L.: Predictable Problems of Hospitalized Adolescents. *Amer. J. Nurs.* 69(3):525–8 (Mar. 69).

    Case study shows how nursing interventions based on a knowledge of basic needs and adolescent development could have averted or minimized serious problems of 19-year-old in cervical traction.

36. Nassen, Andrea: Arteriovenous Shunt Implantation—An Adolescent's Perception and Response. *Amer. J. Nurs.* 70(10):2171–6 (Oct. 70).

    Case study exploring the hypothesis that a patient's psychological adjustment to an arteriovenous shunt depends upon his perception of the effect on his body image, and upon the assistance received in coping with the emotional difficulties experienced.

37. Newton, M., and Folta, J.: Hospital Food Can Help or Hinder Care. *Amer. J. Nurs.* 67(1):112–3 (Jan. 67).

    Describes relationship between patients' values and cultural patterns and the food in a hospital setting. Includes many practical suggestions to help meet the ethnic, social, and psychological needs of patients.

38. Ujhely, Gertrud: Two Types of Problem Patients. *Nursing '76* 6:64–7 (May 76).

    Explores the behavior of a patient who is uncooperative and a patient who gets too personal from the perspective of unmet safety and security needs.

Chapter 5: THE PATIENT'S NEED AND RIGHT TO KNOW

39. Beaumont, E., and Wiley, L., eds.: Home-visit Programs Relieve Adult Fears, Too. *Nursing '74* 4:34–5 (Jan. 74).

    Short article describes a Canadian home-visit program that helps prepare women for surgery and relieves apprehension.

40. Christman, Luther: Assisting the Patient to Learn the "Patient Role." *J. Nurs. Educ.* 6:17–21 (Apr. 67).

    Covers wide range of teaching that need be done before patient can fully participate in all aspects of his care, including evaluation of care received from each member of health care team.

41. Jones, Barbara: Inside the Coronary Care Unit—the Patient and His Responses. *Amer. J. Nurs.* 67(11):2313–20 (Nov. 67).

    Specific, comprehensive description of what coronary patients and their families want, need, feel, and fear. Content generalizable to other critical care units.

42. Kelly, Lucie Young: The Patient's Right to Know. *Nurs. Outlook* 24(1):26–32 (Jan. 76).

Describes increasing legal support for patient's right to know. Discusses attitudes of physicians, informed consent, patient's right of access to his chart, and implications for nursing practice. Gives 26 references.

43. Kelly, Sister Patricia: Diagnostic Tests: What Should We Tell the Patient? *Nursing '74* 4:15–6 (Dec. 74).

Advocates a full explanation to patient about all tests. Includes seven specific guidelines for explaining diagnostic tests.

44. Luciano, K., and Shumsky, C. J.: Pediatric Procedures: The Explanation Should Always Come First. *Nursing '75* 5:49–50, 52 (Jan. 75).

Discounts three reasons for omitting explanations to children. Gives ways to obtain cooperation of pediatricians, describes approaches and techniques appropriate to four age groups, and gives specific tips for interactions with parents.

45. Luckmann, J., and Sorenson, K. C.: The "Sick Role," Chap. 12 in *Medical-Surgical Nursing—A Psychophysiologic Approach.* Philadelphia, W. B. Saunders Company, 1974, pp. 74–5.

Discusses four major aspects of the sick role and indicates that a patient who does not behave as expected is disturbing to health care workers.

46. Prsala, Helena: Admission Unit Dispels Fear of Surgery. *Can. Nurse* 70(12):24–6 (Dec. 74).

Describes effects of patient's four-to-five-hour stay in admission unit where preoperative teaching is one of the planned activities. Bibliography.

47. Robinson, Lisa: Sick Doctors and Nurses Are Sick Human Beings. *Amer. J. Nurs.* 71(9):1728–9 (Sept. 71).

Short case study of nurse who was overwhelmed by illness and was unable to handle all the information she asked for and received.

Chapter 6: TEACHING AND NURSING PROCESS

48. Fuerst, Elinor V., et al.: Description of the Nursing Process System, Chap. 5 in *Fundamentals of Nursing.* 5th ed.; Philadelphia, J. B. Lippincott Company, 1974, pp. 49–54.

Brief introduction to general system theory and nursing process. References included.

49. Gebbie, K., and Lavin, M. A.: Classifying Nursing Diagnoses. *Amer. J. Nurs.* 74(2):250–3 (Feb. 74).

Describes process used by First National Conference on the Classification of Nursing Diagnoses in 1973. Gives tentative list of nursing diagnoses. Describes way in which all nurses can participate in development of classifications.

50. Gordon, Marjory: Nursing Diagnoses and the Diagnostic Process. *Amer. J. Nurs.* 76(8):1298–1300 (Aug. 76).

Describes the Problem–Etiology–Signs/Symptoms (PES) format. Urges nurses to begin to describe the health problems they treat. Differentiates between medical and nursing diagnoses. Nine references.

51. Little, D. E., and Carnevali, D. L.: *Nursing Care Planning.* 2nd ed.; Philadelphia, J. B. Lippincott Company, 1976, Chap. 2, pp. 11–21.

Overview of nursing process, outline of steps and detailed illustration of the clinical application. Discusses relationship between knowledge and each step of the process.

52. Mundinger, M., and Jauron, G.: Developing a Nursing Diagnosis. *Nurs. Outlook* 23 (2):94–8 (Feb. 75).

Experiences of primary nurses in developing a classification system—describes results of a demonstration project, and problems of wording and using diagnoses. Eleven references.

53. Roy, Sister Callista: A Diagnostic Classification System for Nursing. *Nurs. Outlook* 23 (2):90–4 (Feb. 75).

Gives rationale for developing a classification system, rules of categorization, and implications of a system for nursing practice, education, and research. Thirteen references.

Chapter 7: ASSESSMENT OF THE LEARNER

54. Friedland, Geanne: Learning Behaviors of a Preadolescent with Diabetes. *Amer. J. Nurs.* 76(1):59–61 (Jan. 76).

Analyzes the learning behaviors (rote, concrete, and abstract) of an 11-year-old boy in terms of Piaget's theory and describes implications for teaching.

55. Haferkorn, Virginia: Assessing Individual Learning Needs as a Basis for Patient Teaching. *Nurs. Clin. North Am.* 6(1):199–209 (Mar. 71).

Describes general aspects of assessment with specific attention to patient with a myocardial infarction. Gives example of turning point in patient's "readiness."

56. Keeling, Betty L.: Making the Most of the First Home Visit. *Nursing '78* 8:24–8 (Mar. 78).

Describes in detail the wealth of information that can be gained during the first home visit while making the initial assessment of the patient.

57. Kratzer, Joan B.: What Does Your Patient Need to Know? *Nursing '77* 7:82, 84 (Dec. 77).
Describes a four-page *Patient Education Assessment Teaching Plan* used to guide the initial interview, provide a teaching outline, and serve as a permanent record of patient education. Emphasis of article is on assessment.

58. Luckmann, J., and Sorenson, K. C.: Reactions to the Confirmation of Illness, Chap. 10 in *Medical-Surgical Nursing—A Psychophysiologic Approach*. Philadelphia, W. B. Saunders Company, 1974, pp. 64–9.
Describes four general factors that influence a person's reaction to illness. Also discusses 12 specific reactions to diagnosis and state of illness. Important data for assessment of learner.

59. Luckmann, J. and Sorenson, K. C.: Recognizing the Need for Medical Attention, Chap. 9 in *Medical-Surgical Nursing—A Psychophysiologic Approach*. Philadelphia, W. B. Saunders Company, 1974, pp. 61–3.
Describes seven reasons why people do not readily seek medical attention promptly. Also discusses reasons for seeking medical care more often than necessary. This information is needed for adequate assessment of patient.

60. Merkatz, R., et al.: Preoperative Teaching for Gynecologic Patients. *Amer. J. Nurs.* 74(6):1072–4 (June 74).
Describes use of group sessions for preoperative teaching with emphasis on clues that indicate need for individual or additional teaching.

61. Natalini, John: The Human Body as a Biological Clock. *Amer. J. Nurs.* 77:1130–2 (July 77).
An overview of biorhythms with examples of effects and implications for nursing and chronopharmacology. Extensive references with addresses for additional readings.

62. Roznoy, Melinda: The Young Adult: Taking a Sexual History. *Amer. J. Nurs.* 76(8):1279–82 (Aug. 76).
Presents philosophy and process of taking a sexual history with emphasis on purposes of acquiring baseline data, providing education when indicated, and providing anticipatory guidance. Discusses sexuality and the health of families.

Chapter 8: ASSESSMENT OF READINESS TO LEARN

63. Boisvert, Cecile: Convalescence Following Coronary Surgery: A Group Experience. *Can. Nurse* 72(11):26–7 (Nov. 76).

    Study reveals that patients were more receptive to information *after* they returned home. Identifies 11 main concerns that indicate that readiness to learn is high during convalescence.

64. Graham, Lois E.: Patients' Perceptions in the CCU. *Amer. J. Nurs.* 69(9):1921–2 (Sept. 69).

    Study indicates that, for a variety of reasons, patients could recall very little of the information that nurses state was given in the coronary care unit, and that it must be repeated following the acute phase of illness.

65. Laird, Mona: Techniques for Teaching Pre- and Postoperative Patients. *Amer. J. Nurs.* 75(8):1338–40 (Aug. 75).

    A surgical nurse practitioner describes content of pre- and postoperative teaching and discusses overt and covert behavior that indicates the patient is not ready to learn.

66. Stewart, Ruth F.: Education for Health Maintenance. *Occup. Health Nurs.* (NY) 22:14–7 (June 74).

    Discusses group membership as a motivating factor for learning in an industrial setting. Describes role and effect of the informal group leaders.

Chapter 9: ASSESSMENT OF THE TEACHER

67. Stanley, Linda: Does Your Own Body Image Hurt Patient Care? *RN* 40:50–3 (Dec. 77).

    Three psychiatric nurses discuss ways to work through your feelings and ways to help patients cope with deformity or disfigurement. Patient teaching not emphasized, but content is applicable.

Chapter 10: ASSESSMENT OF THE TEACHING SITUATION

68. Aeschliman, Dorothy: Guidelines for Cross-Cultural Health Programs. *Nurs. Outlook* 21(10):660–3 (Oct. 73).

    Gives 10 basic, specific, and practical guidelines for establishing a health program for persons of a different culture. Based on experiences of Project Hope Nurses.

69. Directory of 100 Organizations to Contact for Free or Low-Cost Professional Materials. *Nursing '76* 6:60A–60H (Sept. 76).

    Includes material for self-study, continuing education, or general inservice programs. Printed materials cost under $5, AV materials rent for $20 or less and sell for $50 or less.

70. Fralic, Maryann F.: Developing a Viable Inpatient Education Program—A Nursing Director's Perspective. *J. Nurs. Admin.* 76:30–6 (Sept. 76).

    Describes a comprehensive teaching program that is responsive to patient needs, satisfying to staff, and notably cost-effective. Gives specific protocols for diabetic, ostomy, and cardiac patients.

71. Fuhrer, L., and Bernstein, R.: Making Patient Education a Part of Patient Care. *Amer. J. Nurs.* 76:1798–9 (Nov. 76).

    Account of two nurses, employed to foster patient education, who set up a resource group of interested nurses who not only teach patients but teach other nurses. Resource nurses for orthopedics, psychiatry, colostomy, stroke rehabilitation, mastectomy, and urology/gynecology were included.

72. Nordberg, B., and King, L.: Third Party Payment for Patient Education. *Nurs. Digest* 8:32–4 (Spring 78).

    Very practical guide for persons trying to initiate payment arrangements for patient education. Describes preparation of the proposal and strategies for dealing with insurance carriers.

73. Porter, Sharon F.: Diabetic Education: Role for the Inservice Instructor. *Supervisor Nurse* 8:49–53 (May 77).

    Detailed account of how a high caliber of patient education can be achieved by a technical nurse if proper support system is provided (multidisciplinary committee, adequate material and time).

74. Stein, Terry: Establishing Prenatal Classes in a Small Community—Overcoming the Opposition. *JOGN Nurs.* 2:44–8 (Sept.–Oct. 73).

    Explores relationships within community system that facilitated or hindered the development of prenatal classes. Resources and class outline are included.

75. Stevens, P., and Conkling, V.: We Teach Breast Self-Examination to Hospital Patients. *RN* 77:25–31 (Jan. 77).

    Over 8000 female patients in one hospital have been taught BSE as a result of support of the hospital, local cancer society, and staff nurses.

76. Valentine, Lois R.: Self-Care through Group Learning. *Amer. J. Nurs.* 70(10):2140–2 (Oct. 70).

    A professional team representing medicine, nursing, physical medicine, occupational therapy, social service, and dietary presents eight classes for arthritic patients. Content for each class is included.

77. Wood, M. Marian: 300 Valuable Booklets to Give to Patients and their Families: A Source Guide. Part I (A–L) *Nursing '74* 4:43–50 (Apr. 74). Part II (M–Z) *Nursing '74* 4:59–66 (May 74).

Includes description, price (if any), and ordering information for each booklet or pamphlet.

78. Woske, M., and Kratzer, J.: C.T.—Cardiac Teaching: Preparing the Patient for a Different Life. *Nursing* '77 7:25–6 (May 77).

Describes preparation of Cardiac Teaching nurses as well as development of program. Includes methods of teaching, instructional materials, and evaluation methods. Description is detailed and comprehensive.

Chapters 11 and 12: OBJECTIVES AND DOMAINS OF LEARNING

79. Anderson, M. I.: Development of Outcome Criteria for the Patient with Congestive Heart Failure. *Nurs. Clin. North Am.* 9(2):349–58 (June 74).

Detailed presentation of outcome criteria and their potential usefulness as a teaching tool in patient education.

80. Dicken, Annette: Why Patients Should Plan their Own Recovery. *RN* 41:52–5 (Mar. 78).

Describes relationships of goal setting to motivation, and explains how patient goal setting works in clinical situations.

81. Gronlund, Norman E.: *Stating Objectives for Classroom Instruction.* 2nd ed.; New York, The Macmillan Company, 1978, 74 pages.

82. McFarlane, J., and Hames, C. C.: Children with Diabetes Learning Self-Care in Camp. *Amer. J. Nurs.* 73(8):1362–5 (Aug. 73).

Two case studies illustrate the use of behavioral objectives in teaching children to independently care for their diabetes.

Chapter 13: SELECTION OF CONTENT AND METHOD

83. Aiken, Linda H.: Patient Problems Are Problems in Learning. *Amer. J. Nurs.* 70(9):1916–8 (Sept. 70).

Emphasizes need for assessment of patient problems before to choosing a method of teaching. Brief description of systematic desensitization and behavior modification, applied to two patient situations.

84. Altshuler, Anne, et al.: Even Children Can Learn to Do Clean Self-Catheterization. *Amer. J. Nurs.* 77:97–101 (Jan. 77).

Illustrates how research can influence both the content and methods of patient teaching. Includes underlying theory and detailed explanation of how to teach self-catheterization to children.

85. Baden, Catherine A.: Teaching the Coronary Patient and His Family. *Nurs. Clin. North Am.* 7(3):563–71 (Sept. 72).

Describes development of posthospital education program, since teaching cannot be accomplished adequately during hospital stay. Includes objectives of program and course content.

86. Eddy, Mary E.: Teaching Patients with Peripheral Vascular Disease. *Nurs. Clin. North Am.* 12(1):151–9 (Mar. 77).
   Illustrates how essential content about disease can be integrated with needs and problems of learner to give learning goals. Factors that affect the patient's ability to learn are discussed.

87. Larter, Mariella H.: "M.I. Wives" Need You. *RN* 39:44–8 (Aug. 76).
   Describes a study to determine the kind of help needed and the ways in which nurses can help. The same method is applicable to other diseases or conditions.

88. Long, Madeleine, et al.: Hypertension: What Patients Need to Know. *Amer. J. Nurs.* 76(5):765–70 (May 76).
   Contains much information about disease, drugs, and other aspects of therapy. Also, detailed description of content for patient teaching.

89. Mitchell, Ellen: Protocol for Teaching Hypertensive Patients. *Amer. J. Nurs.* 77:808–9 (May 77).
   An example of a format for patient teaching. Content and method are outlined in steps and substeps that are easy to follow and likely to give consistent results. Applicable to many other areas of patient teaching.

90. Moore, K., and Maschak, B. J.: How Patient Education Can Reduce the Risks of Anticoagulant Therapy. *Nursing '77* 7:25–9 (Sept. 77).
   Stresses importance of good knowledge of disease before trying to teach. Also the importance of teaching patient to use acquired information. Includes details of content to be taught.

91. Moyer, P. J., and Conover, B. J.: The Now Style of Campus Nursing. *Amer. J. Nurs.* 70(9):1900–3 (Sept. 70).
   Graphic example of how the selection of both content and method of teaching depends upon an assessment of the learners.

92. Owen, Bernice D.: The Middle Years: Coping With Chronic Illness. *Amer. J. Nurs.* 75(6):1016–8 (June 75).
   Presents examples of content arising from the needs of the learner and his family.

93. Williams, Barbara P.: The Burned Patient's Need for Teaching. *Nurs. Clin. North Amer.* 6(4):615–9, 637–8 (Dec. 71).
   Explains how content for teaching is derived from nurse's knowledge of problems common to burn patients as well as from patient's anticipation of how his way of living may change as a result of being burned.

Chapter 14: METHODS OF TEACHING

94. Baker, Dorothy: Hyperalimentation at Home. *Amer. J. Nurs.* 74(10):1826–9 (Oct. 74).

Nurse practitioner, in consultation with professional resource persons, proves that hyperalimentation therapy can be done at home without expensive equipment or specialized medical resources. Includes details of problems and their solutions.

95. Conte, Andrea, et al.: Group Work with Hypertensive Patients. *Amer. J. Nurs.* 74(5):910–2 (May 74).

Useful description of teaching techniques, ways of evaluating learning, and benefits to patients. Content not limited to hypertension; applicable to other types of patient groups.

96. D'Afflitti, J. G., and Swanson, D.: Group Sessions for the Wives of Home-Hemodialysis Patients. *Amer. J. Nurs.* 75(4):633–5 (Apr. 75).

A home training program uses group sessions to provide emotional support for wives. Nondirective group leaders encouraged expression of anger, guilt, helplessness, and other feelings that could interfere with home dialysis.

97. Deberry, Pauline, et al.: Teaching Cardiac Patients to Manage Medications. *Amer. J. Nurs.* 75(12):2191–3 (Dec. 75).

Discusses specific methods of teaching and shows relationship between evaluation of learning and the selection or modification of teaching strategies.

98. Healy, Kathryn M.: A Pre-operative Patient Teaching Program. *AORN J* 10:37–43 (Oct. 69).

Describes the use of a pre-op teaching aid called "Color Me Green," written in Spanish and English. Heavy emphasis upon need to assess the learner.

99. McClure, J. J., and Ryburn, A. C.: Care-by-Parent Unit. *Amer. J. Nurs.* 69(10):2148–52 (Oct. 69).

Describes the unique opportunities for teaching in an experimental unit for children who do not need full-time professional supervision. Mentions a variety of teaching techniques.

100. Moore, Karen, et al.: The Joy of Sex after a Heart Attack. *Nursing '77* 7:53–5 (June 77).

Three nurses prepare a 12-page illustrated booklet titled *The Cardiac Patient and Sex.* The role and uses of printed material in patient teaching are discussed.

101. Nunnally, Dianne M.: A New Approach to Helping Mothers Breastfeed. *JOGN Nurs.* 3(4):34—5 (July—Aug. 74).

    Demonstrates that breastfeeding can be successfully taught in a class that combines instruction in theory with actual practice in feeding babies. Includes list of teaching aids.

102. Park, Sherry: Preoperative "Teach-in." *Can. Nurse* 68:38—9 (Oct. 72).

    Describes use of daily group sessions to prepare patients for surgery, followed by specific or individual teaching. Includes discussion of planning and content.

103. Patterson, K., and Pomeroy, M.: Nursing Care Begins after Death When the Disease Is: Sudden Infant Death Syndrome. *Nursing '74* 4:85—8 (May 74).

    Illustrates the effective use of questions by nurse in helping parents to talk about and learn about SIDS. Process applicable to other situations involving grief and guilt.

104. Raynolds, Nancy: Teaching Parents Home Care after Surgery for Scoliosis. *Amer. J. Nurs.* 74(6):1090—2 (June 74).

    Describes a three-day, live-in program for parents. Discusses content, methods, of teaching and benefits to patient and family.

105. Waterson, Marian: Teaching Your Patients Postural Drainage. *Nursing '78* 8:51—3 (Mar. 78).

    Describes the *process* of teaching postural drainage as well as the content. Includes a Patient Teaching Aid, which can be photocopied, and a check list of Do's and Don't's. Process is applicable to other conditions.

106. Williamson, K. C., and McCary, N.: Putting Together a Patient Education Program That Works. *RN* 40:53—5 (Nov, 77).

    Describes the use of "teaching baskets," which hold everything the nurse needs to help patient understand a treatment regimen. Each basket contains teaching guides for nurse and AV aids for patient. Details of contents and use of baskets are included.

Chapter 15: USE OF AUDIOVISUAL MATERIALS

107. Brown, James, et al.: *AV Instruction—Technology, Media and Methods.* 4th ed.; New York, McGraw-Hill Book Company, 1973, 584 pages.

    Comprehensive textbook focusing upon media in relation to the activity of learning. Includes theoretical and practical considerations of selecting, using, producing, and evaluating educational media.

108. Brown, J. W., and Lewis, R. B.: *AV Instructional Technology Manual for Independent Study.* 4th ed.; New York, McGraw-Hill Book Company, 1973, 184 pages.

    Self-study manual correlated with the textbook listed above. Designed to facilitate the use of AV equipment and development of materials. Extensive references and sources for AV materials.

109. Gustafson, Marilyne B.: The Blackboard Chalkboard Revisited. *Supervisor Nurse* 8:57, 59, 61 (May 77).

    Detailed and comprehensive guide for using a chalkboard. Includes nine suggestions to maximize use and five variations in use. References list sources of information related to use of puzzles and games.

Chapter 16: SELECTED ASPECTS OF INSTRUCTION

Feedback

110. Ginott, Haim G.: New Ways of Praise and Criticism, Chap. 2 in *Between Parent and Child.* New York, The Macmillan Company, 1965, pp. 37–52.

    Describes, very simply, how to praise or criticize a person's behavior without labeling his personality.

111. Koscel, Jessie: How Patients Use a Logbook. *Amer. J. Nurs.* 74(7):1307 (July 74).

    Describes how women in a comprehensive alcoholism program write their own daily reports. Similar feedback from patients in other types of units could be feasible.

112. Kramer, M., and Schmalenberg, C.: Constructive Feedback. *Nursing '77* 7:102, 104, 106 (Nov. 77).

    Gives specific, practical ways to exchange constructive feedback with co-workers. Readily applicable to patient teaching as well as to non-nursing situations.

113. Luckmann, J., and Sorenson, K. C.: Man Struggles to Maintain a State of Balance, Chapter 3 in *Medical-Surgical Nursing—A Phychophysiologic Approach.* Philadelphia, W. B. Saunders Company, 1974, pp. 17–25.

    Describes homeostatic mechanisms, and explains positive and negative feedback with reference to physiology. Many references.

Reward and Reinforcement

114. Carruth, Beatrice F.: Modifying Behavior through Social Learning. *Amer. J. Nurs.* 76:1804–6 (Nov. 76).

Describes how graduate students learned to use reinforcement to treat disturbed children and adult psychiatric patients. Gives overview of social learning theory (part of behavior modification).

115. Pace, J. Blair: Helping Patients Overcome the Disabling Effects of Chronic Pain. *Nursing '77* 7:38–43 (July 77).

Detailed description of reinforcement as a means to reprogram pain behavior and establish desirable behaviors. Numerous examples make the material practical and useful.

116. Schwartz, M., and White, M.: Motivating Clinic Patients. *Supervisor Nurse* 8:48–9 (Oct. 77).

Study compares the effectiveness of social reinforcement versus material reward ($20) in motivating patients to keep clinic appointment.

117. Whitman, H., and Lukes, S.: Behavior Modification for Terminally Ill Patients. *Amer. J. Nurs.* 75(1):98–101 (Jan. 75).

Describes the process and guidelines for using behavior modification to help patients alter maladaptive behavior, begin realistic problem solving, and communicate more effectively with families and staff.

Language

118. Cosper, Bonnie: How Well Do Patients Understand Hospital Jargon? *Amer. J. Nurs.* 77(12):1932–4 (Dec. 77).

Study indicates considerable lack of understanding of commonly used hospital words. Includes four recommendations to reduce patient anxiety and promote understanding.

119. Smith, Elaine C.: Are You Really Communicating? *Amer. J. Nurs.* 77(12):1966–8 (Dec. 77).

Study indicates that school children (grades three to five) attach inaccurate and idiosyncratic meanings to words, and that they have meager knowledge about the human body. Emphasizes need for nurse to adapt her verbal messages to need and level of understanding.

Chapter 17: EVALUATION AND PATIENT TEACHING

120. Allendorf, E. E., and Keegan, M. H.: Teaching Patients about Nitroglycerin. *Amer. J. Nurs.* 75(7):1168–70 (July 75).

Twenty patients were interviewed and found to lack enough knowledge about nitroglycerin to use it safely and effectively. Concise and comprehensive guidelines for teaching patients and details of the evaluation are included.

121. Eaton, Sharon et al.: Discussion Stoppers in Teaching. *Nurs. Outlook* 25:578–83 (Sept. 77).

Describes eleven examples of teacher behaviors that tend to stop or disrupt discussion. Suggestions for changing these behaviors are included.

122. Healy, Kathryn M.: Does Preoperative Instruction Make a Difference? *Amer. J. Nurs.* 68 (1):62–7 (Jan. 68).

Describes the criteria used to evaluate the effectiveness of preoperative teaching. Content and method of instruction are described in detail.

123. Jessop, Penny: Stepping Stones: A Road to Coronary Rehabilitation Programs. *Can. Nurse* 72(11):18–21 (Nov. 76).

Includes development of programs and a sample patient assessment form. Comprehensive and detailed presentation on methods of evaluation, including criteria, can serve as model for evaluation in other patient teaching situations.

124. Kos, B., and Culbert, P.: Teaching Patients about Pacemakers. *Amer. J. Nurs.* 71(3):523–7 (Mar. 71).

Comprehensive description of program, including assessment of learning. Discusses use of pre- and post tests, a questionnaire to determine application of knowledge to daily life, and a description of behaviors that indicate motivation.

125. Leary, Jean A., et al.: Self-administered Medications. *Amer. J. Nurs.* 71(6):1193–4 (June 71).

Describes a way to evaluate patients' knowledge of their medications, describes the findings, and examines the role of nurses in teaching about medications.

126. Salzer, Joan E.: Classes to Improve Diabetic Self-care. *Amer. J. Nurs.* 75(8):1324–6 (Aug. 75).

Describes how a nurse planned, conducted, and evaluated a series of three classes. Questionnaires were sent one month after classes and again after one year. Results indicated increased ability to care for self.

127. Watkins, J. D., and Moss, F. T.: Confusion in the Management of Diabetes. *Amer. J. Nurs.* 69(3):521–4 (Mar. 69).

Documents with examples the need for periodic evaluation of the patients' management in order to ascertain need for further teaching to compensate for changes in patients' life and condition.

APPENDIX A

Evaluation of Instructional Materials

Title _____
Producer _____
Distributor or source_____
Type: _____ 16mm Film   _____ Audio tape (reel)
       _____ 8mm Film loop   _____ Audio tape (cassette)
       _____ Filmstrip   _____ Video tape
       _____ 35mm slides   _____ Video tape (cassette)
       _____ Record   _____ Programmed text
       _____ Transparency   Other (write in) _____
Date produced _____ Running time: ____ Black & white: ____ Color: ____
Evaluator: Name _____ Date _____
          Position (check one): Staff nurse ____ Patient educator ____
          Patient _____ Age ____ Family member_____
          Other (write in)_____
1. Brief description of content (use other side if necessary):

2. Level of material presented: ____ beginning ____ intermediate
                                              ____ advanced
3. Suggested or possible uses: ____ introduce a subject;
   ____ stimulate discussion; ____ present essential information;
   ____ review; ____ other:_____
4. Personal opinion: ____ interesting; ____ dull; ____ repetetive;
   ____ other (write in)_____

5. Prerequisite knowledge (list or describe):
   essential for understanding:

   helpful for understanding:

6. Outstanding feature(s):

7. Accuracy of information presented:

8. Currency of information presented:

9. Depth of coverage:

10. Technical qualities:
    a) Sound track: diction _____
                     volume _____
                     pacing _____
    b) Visual aspects: quality of photography _____
       Quality of diagrams, charts, etc. _____
    c) Synchronization of sound and visual aspects: _____
11. Educational aspects:
    Pacing of presentation: _____
    Appropriate selection of visual material (live model, line drawing,
    real situation, animation, etc.) _____
    Other: _____
12. Additional comments:

APPENDIX B

Selection of Audiovisual Materials

AUDIOVISUAL MATERIALS FROM WHICH A SELECTION MAY BE MADE:

Blackboard	Audiotapes	Pamphlets
Flannel board	Videotapes	Photographs
Posters, charts	Live television	Diagram
Scale models	Telelecture	Records
Slides	Computers	Duplicated "handouts"
Filmstrips	Textbooks	Actual objects (e.g., pacemaker)
Film loops	Printed programs	Patients
16mm film	Magazines	Transparencies

FACTORS THAT INFLUENCE THE SELECTION AND USE OF AUDIOVISUAL MATERIALS:

1. Material to be taught
   Does it involve abstract concepts, application of principles, motor skills, extensive practice, etc.?
   How frequently must it be presented? Frequently enough to justify a large expenditure of funds? How rapidly will the content become outdated?

2. Objectives
   What do you expect to accomplish by using AV materials?

3. Trends in education
   What is happening in general education? How can nursing benefit from research in general education regarding the use of AV materials?

4. Staff

What is the attitude of the staff toward the use of AV materials?

What skills does the staff have regarding the use of AV materials?

What kind of an inservice program may be needed?

If a major expenditure is being considered, will enough of the staff use the facilities as a method of teaching their own content to justify the expense?

5. Space

Is there adequate space for safe storage of expensive materials and equipment?

Is there space for teaching with AV materials and for any practice that may be essential to certain units?

6. Accessibility

Who will schedule the use of major pieces of equipment?

Who will catalogue AV materials?

Who will check these materials in and out?

Will these materials (and space) be available evenings and weekends?

7. Equipment (hardware)

How expensive are the projectors, cameras, and other items that you are considering?

What are the problems of maintenance and repair for each piece of equipment?

How difficult is it to operate the equipment?

8. Teaching materials (software)

What film loops, slides, videotapes are available?

What materials will be available?

Could you make your own materials?

Are they easy to use?

Are they durable enough for use?

For each specific item (film loop, filmstrips, etc.) that you preview or consider using:

By whom was it prepared?

For whom was it prepared?

Does it accomplish its stated objective?

Will it contribute to your objectives?

Will its use be effective enough to justify the expense?

Are study guides and teachers' manuals available?

9. Motor skills
   Does the content to be taught require a medium that will permit action, such as film or videotape

   or

   Can the skill be analyzed and broken down into a series of still photographs or slides?
   Would a multimedia approach be desirable?
   (Examples—Film loop to orient to the entire procedure, following with slides or photographs of difficult parts.

   or

   A videotape of procedure followed by film loop with closeups of critical points.)
10. Optimal use
    Could the materials be used for more than one level of learner? (E.g.: using a sequence of slides for patients, families, and groups of learners in the community by varying the narration that accompanies it.)
11. What AV resources are available within the agency and community?

Index